Reference Manual for Humanitarian Health Professionals

David A. Bradt • Christina M. Drummond

Reference Manual for Humanitarian Health Professionals

Missioncraft in Disaster Relief® Series

6th Edition

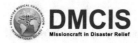

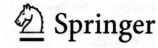

David A. Bradt, MD, MPH, FACEP, FACEM,
FAFPHM, DTM&H
Washington, DC
USA

Christina M. Drummond, AM, MBBS,
DObst(RCOG), DTM&H, FRACP, MPH, MAE,
FAFPHM
Melbourne
Australia

The Work has been published previously as first (2011), second (2013), third (2014), fourth (2015), and fifth (2016) editions by Disaster Medical Coordination International Society (DMCIS) with the title Missioncraft in Disaster Relief Operations -- A Field Manual for Medical Personnel (self-published by the Society)

ISBN 978-3-030-09919-0   ISBN 978-3-319-69871-7   (eBook)
https://doi.org/10.1007/978-3-319-69871-7

Printed on acid-free paper

This Springer imprint is published by Springer Nature, under the registered company Springer International Publishing AG
The registered company address is: Gewerbestrasse 11, 6330 Cham, Switzerland

This Reference Manual is dedicated to the humanitarian aid workers, including local staff, who have lost their lives serving others and to those who labor in the field with little safety, security, comfort, or thanks.

Acknowledgments

We wish to acknowledge the mentors, teachers, and colleagues who have taught us our craft. These black belt operators have collectively saved the lives of countless thousands of people and helped save ours as well. We are eternally in their debt.

Field
- Tom Durant*—Cambodia, Zaire, Bosnia, Macedonia
- Bob Brenner—Pakistan, Laos, Peru
- Peter Galpin—places dark and scary
- Judy Lee—USA
- Luis Jorge Perez—Indonesia, India
- Pino Annunziata—Indonesia, Tunisia
- Johanna Larusdottir—India, Sri Lanka
- Eigil Sorensen—Indonesia, India
- Kate Farnsworth—Sudan
- Andre Kisselev—Zaire
- Keith Bentley—Indonesia
- Tom Dolan—Indonesia
- Nawal Osman—Sudan
- Haider Abu Ahmed—Sudan
- AK Siddique—Bangladesh
- Marguerite Ryle*—USA
- Jim Ellis*—Cambodia

Headquarters of governmental, nongovernmental, Red Cross, and UN organizations
(Individuals are identified with their institutional affiliation during formative periods of interaction with the authors. Cited affiliations are not necessarily current.)
- Skip Burkle—Harvard Humanitarian Initiative
- Tim Baker*—Johns Hopkins University School of Public Health
- Sue Baker—Johns Hopkins University School of Public Health
- Allen Yung*—Fairfield Infectious Diseases Hospital
- Pierre Perrin—International Committee of the Red Cross
- Rudi Coninx—International Committee of the Red Cross
- Claude de Ville de Goyet—Pan-American Health Organization
- Helene Monteil—American Red Cross International Services
- Jorge Castilla—World Health Organization
- Fred Cuny*—Intertech
- Peter Wallis—USAID Office of US Foreign Disaster Assistance
- Mike VanRooyen—Johns Hopkins University School of Medicine

*   In memoriam

We are grateful to the following foundations and societies for their assistance during critical phases of this work:

Rockefeller Foundation

John Simon Guggenheim Memorial Foundation

Australasian Society for Infectious Diseases

We thank Peter Galpin, Amanda Norton, and Jonathan Robinson of the Disaster Medical Coordination International Society for their guidance, encouragement, and enduring support.

David A. Bradt   Christina M. Drummond
Washington, DC, USA   Melbourne, Australia

Contents

Introduction

Reference Manual for Humanitarian Health Professionals—Missioncraft in Disaster Relief is written for humanitarian health professionals who take responsibility for health outcomes of disaster-affected populations.

- *Missioncraft* is the art and science of preparing and conducting effective field operations.
- *Disaster* is defined qualitatively as a natural or man-made phenomenon, which produces large-scale disruption of the normal healthcare system, presents immediate threat to public health, and requires external assistance for response. Quantitative definitions go beyond the scope of this *Manual*.
- *Relief* operations are humanitarian activities undertaken in the acute aftermath of sudden-onset disasters, as well as in the protracted aftermath of complex disasters. The goal is to do the most good for the most people and thereby enable a return to marginal self-sufficiency. Relief operations pursue this goal by incremental objectives in saving lives, alleviating suffering, and reducing the impact of disaster. Activities that do not address these objectives are noncontributory.

Disasters do terrible things to people and societies. Beyond their immediate impacts, disasters set back development. In that context, approximately a third of the world's population may be considered developmentally denied by disasters each decade. However, disasters are opportunities to place vulnerable populations at the center of relief, recovery, and development agendas.

The goal of the *Manual* is to help standardize and improve the professional practice of humanitarian health specialists—managers, educators, researchers, and practitioners. Humanitarian health professionals require immediate, accessible, and authoritative technical information derived from interdisciplinary, interagency, and international best practices in core domains of disaster health. They are frequently burdened with data overload, information poverty, and the relentless pace of just-in-time decision-making. They need a rich, portable fund of knowledge and state-of-the-art tools that enable them to cross professional boundaries as well as international ones. This *Manual* focuses on their needs. Intended attributes of the *Manual* are conceptual rigor as well as ease of application. Conceptual rigor means a consistent approach to acquiring, analyzing, and reporting disaster data. Ease of application means simple and versatile instruments for multitasking health professionals working under tight deadlines in urgent settings.

Conceptual Frameworks

This *Manual* is informed by two conceptual frameworks—technical domains in disaster health (Fig. 1) and management priorities (Fig. 2).

Technical Domains

Disaster relief operations comprise a multidisciplinary body of knowledge. Figure 1 illustrates a basic conceptual framework for disaster health. Competencies in clinical medicine, public health, and disaster management are fundamental. While the three core disciplines do not encompass all disciplines relevant to disaster health—engineering, economics, sociology, and religion among those unmentioned—they do encompass essential scientific expertise required in the health sector. Education and training, field practice, and continuing professional development all derive from a clear understanding of these different domains.

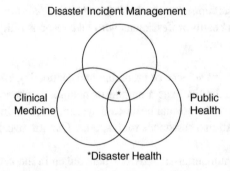

Fig. 1 Technical domains in disaster health

Management Priorities

Dating from pioneering work of UNHCR in the 1980s, the relative impact of different disaster relief interventions has been generally appreciated for over 30 years. Security stabilization in the humanitarian space is fundamental to all sustainable health interventions. Environmental health is a major determinant of health status where deficiencies may have consequences that overwhelm the public health and clinical resources of the health system. Public health in general and primary prevention in particular are among the most cost-effective interventions in the allied health arsenal. In clinical medicine, community and primary care deliver far more accessible and cost-effective health interventions than does hospital-based referral care. Figure 2 illustrates this hierarchy of management priorities in disaster relief.

The ABCs of disaster health in priority order are security, environmental health, public health, and clinical care. Those interventions which most impact the health status of disaster-affected populations—high leverage interventions—are located at the base of the pyramid. Those interventions which least impact the health status of disaster-affected populations—low

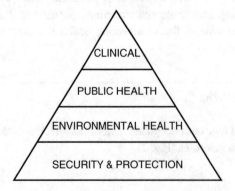

Fig. 2 Management priorities in disaster health

leverage interventions—are located at the apex of the pyramid. Understanding this principle fosters allocative efficiency of relief programs.

The diagram does not predict health interventions in all disaster contexts. For example, transportation disasters may have no security, environmental health, or public health consequences. The relief effort for health professionals may focus almost exclusively on clinical care in the prehospital and hospital settings. However, this *Manual* is purposefully disaster agnostic. Disasters under consideration encompass "all hazards." Just as the ABCs of clinical care provide a consistent, comprehensive, predictable, serially preemptive approach to management of a patient in extremis, so do the ABCs of disaster relief provide a consistent, comprehensive, predictable, serially preemptive approach to management of a population in extremis.

Unfortunately, basic principles are often selectively ignored by many agencies that intervene by mandate and by many clinicians who intervene by invitation. In this context, the *Manual* attempts to foster interdisciplinary, interagency, and international best practices among health personnel. We look forward to an increasing convergence of normative technical practices among career humanitarian health professionals in the future.

Organization of the Manual

The *Manual* provides guidance on key domains of missioncraft—**predeparture preparation, field briefing, field assessment, field recommendations, field reporting, field project and staff management, medical coordination, and reentry**. Each domain is addressed in a dedicated section of the *Manual*. Sections are sequenced in the *Manual* as listed above. This sequence aligns with the chronological order of generic steps in disaster relief operations. Hence, information derived from one section may inform actions in the next section. Individual sections may also be used as needed to address issues spontaneously arising in the field.

Individual sections are organized in the following sequence—**guidance notes, core documents, tools, and technical annexes**.

Guidance Notes present insights to best use of the sections and selected documents under real-time field conditions.

Core Documents are concise, comprehensive data gathering templates. They are self-contained, portable, and formatted for immediate use. The documents are data-dense and written in outline format—hierarchy of I, A, 1, a, (1), (a), (i)—with co-located indicator, black space for field data, and reference benchmark. They are consistently organized in line with the conceptual framework. Overall, the Core Documents function as minimum essential datasets (MEDS). These MEDS enable the user to arrive at an early, accurate picture of the health situation in the field. MEDS are sufficiently detailed to be authoritative, sufficiently brief to be manageable, and sufficiently useful to inform most common decisions made about health programs in the field. It is understood that not all data points, even in a MEDS framework, are needed to inform field decisions. Small amounts of reliable, relevant data will usually suffice.

Tools are documents for additional data capture in specific areas that inform and strengthen the Core Documents. Core Documents occasionally became unwieldy when Tools were integrated directly into them. Hence, Tools are presented here as stand-alone documents, which are particularly useful when tracking unstable field conditions where data are perishable.

Core Documents and Tools are working documents identified in the *Manual* by the section in which they appear.

e.g.:   Document 2.1 refers to the first core document of Section 2.

e.g.:   Tool 3.T2 refers to the second tool of Section 3.

Items in parentheses ( ) are acronyms, indicators, units of measure, reference benchmarks, and/or information sources.

Technical Annexes are repositories of core technical information located in Section 8 of the *Manual*.

Glossaries are placed in the sections of the *Manual* with a high burden of technical abbreviations and acronyms—Section 3 Guidance Notes and Section 8 Annexes 3–7. **Acronyms**, particularly of institutional and bureaucratic origin, are extensively listed in Section 8 Annex 8. **References** are placed at the end of relevant Guidance Notes, Documents, or Annexes. Annexes, in particular, cite selected classic articles in the biomedical literature.

Application

Data are not created equal. Many indicators exist for any given subject, and they have different sources, acquisition methods, availabilities, utilities, costs, and technical limitations. This *Manual* does not detail these issues but rather makes an explicit judgment about indicator usefulness through *de facto* inclusion in datasets. Moreover, providers are not trained equal. We do not explain indicators in this *Manual*. We simply use them as needed to help characterize the professional practice of disaster health specialists.

Medical coordinators may choose to customize the Core Documents with indicators and benchmarks most relevant to their agency. Some programmatic decisions in some specialty areas (e.g., immunization programs, feeding programs) may require additional data gathered through dedicated surveys or disease surveillance beyond the scope of this *Manual*. Where the reader is unfamiliar with elements of documents, tools, and methods in the *Manual*, he is encouraged to simply adopt what appears useful and to ignore the rest. Unless stated otherwise, masculine nouns and pronouns in the *Manual* refer to both genders.

Feedback

Humanitarian health professionals work in donor agencies, academic institutions, think tanks, relief organizations, as well as the "field." The "field" is not the capital city or country office. It is often not even the field office. The "field" is where the beneficiaries are found. Ground truth comes from the deep field. The way to do important work is to work on important things. Humanitarian health professionals undertake important things in urgent settings. They will be the ultimate judges of usefulness of the *Manual*. To that end, feedback from experienced users is welcomed at info@dmcis.org.

Disclaimer

Reference Manual for Humanitarian Health Professionals—Missioncraft in Disaster Relief is written, compiled, and published as a reference source of information for humanitarian health professionals on health sector management in disasters. It is intended to supplement, not replace, specific real-time research into critical disaster and emergency response topics. If you have a specific inquiry that requires up-to-date and authoritative information, you are urged to visit the websites of agencies and professional associations included in this *Reference Manual*. No medical advice is provided or distributed from this *Reference Manual*. Users interested in medical advice or treatment must consult a properly licensed medical practitioner familiar with their health history. Physicians and other healthcare professionals are advised to consult their usual clinical resources before prescribing specific products or drugs to their patients. Any practice described in this *Reference Manual* should be applied by healthcare professionals in accordance with professional judgment and standards of care appropriate for the unique circumstances of each situation they encounter.

Most of the websites cited in this *Reference Manual* are external to the authors and publisher. These external websites are provided as a service and do not imply any official endorsement of or responsibility for the opinions, ideas, content, or products presented on them. The authors and publisher cannot and do not guarantee or warrant that files available for downloading from any website will be free of infection from viruses, worms, Trojan horses, or other code that may manifest contaminating or destructive properties.

Although the authors and publisher undertake reasonable efforts to keep the information contained in this *Reference Manual* accurate, the authors and publisher do not warrant the accuracy, completeness, timeliness, merchantability, or fitness for a particular purpose of the information contained in this *Reference Manual*. The above warranties are the only warranties of any kind either expressed or implied. In no event shall the authors or publisher be liable to you or anyone else for any decision made or action taken by you in reliance on such information. The authors and publisher are not responsible for errors, omissions, or inaccuracies in information of any kind, or for any damage or loss involving clinician users, their patients, or other users, whether direct, indirect, special, incidental, exemplary, or consequential, arising from or caused by use of or reliance upon any information contained in or distributed through this *Reference Manual*.

Pre-Departure Preparation

Contents

Guidance Notes

Disaster may strike without warning, and deployment may come without warning. International deployments may occur with less than 4 hours' notice—although 2–3 days is more common. The humanitarian health professional embraces the burden of continuous readiness. One who waits for activation before preparing for departure is flirting with disaster—whether to himself, his team, or his beneficiaries.

Deployment involves a range of administrative procedures including medical clearance and vaccination, travel planning (visas, tickets, insurance), field level safety and security, in-country transportation and accommodation, staff health and medical evacuation, and administrative support. To this end, pre-departure personal preparation is often perceived as episodic, ad hoc, and exceptional. It should be continuous, iterative, and routine. Detailed core packing and task lists are critical. The burden of compiling such lists has its rewards—decreased packing mistakes, decreased stress, and increased familiarity with the gear. You don't really know your gear until you know its features and faults, and can find it in the dark, in the cold, and in a hurry. Disciplined personal preparation confers this ability upon the provider. Pre-departure team preparation is beyond the scope of this *Manual*.

There are two major domains of preparation—information and personal effects.

Information (Document 1.1)

Information is the most challenging domain to prepare. The time between disaster onset and staff mobilization may be short—hours or days. In that window, information management takes up the bulk of our preparation time with finding, downloading, archiving, transcribing, and analyzing relevant information. There are two major types of information:

1. Country and event-specific information (what happened where)
2. Generic technical reference information (e.g., cholera control guidelines)

© David A. Bradt 2019
D. A. Bradt, C. M. Drummond, *Reference Manual for Humanitarian Health Professionals*,
https://doi.org/10.1007/978-3-319-69871-7_1

Country and Event-Specific Information

The most urgent aspect of information management is compiling country and event-specific information. Building this archive is a mission-specific activity. The process generally begins only after a disaster is declared, and a personal activation is ordered. Time is at a premium. Useful information encompasses at least 6 sub-types—geographic/weather information; situation reports; sociopolitical, consular, & cultural reports; health reports; linguistic information; and administrative information. Due diligence is facilitated by a master list of authoritative websites to visit (web lists) as well as a directory structure in which to archive useful documents (see Document 1.1). UN websites typically reference all UN member states, present a standardized database structure, and offer downloadable pdfs. Disaster response agencies and donors will quickly complicate information management with new websites devoted to the specific disaster. These key new websites must be also archived in one's browser and entered into web lists.

Upon activation for deployment, important documents can be downloaded, stored, skimmed for relevance, and printed for reading on the way. For a sudden-onset natural disaster, the approximate times for selected tasks follow below:

- Data/document downloading from a concise web list—about 1 h
- Data/document archiving (filing soft copy and/or hard copy)—about 1/2 h
- Data/document transcribing on field assessment sheets of Section 3—about 1 h
- Data analysis—about 2 h

Briefing information should also be provided by your sponsoring organization. The yield from this is highly variable. Further details are found in Section 2 Field Briefing.

The key for a medical coordinator is familiarity with selected documents relevant to his practice. Once in the field, production of authoritative, just-in-time information is a hallmark of a competent medical coordinator. A memory stick full of unexamined documents is probably less useful than a simple web browser. And one should not count on reliable internet access in the field post-disaster.

An indicative information packing list follows in this section. It is not intended to be prescriptive. General comments are bulleted below.

- Web lists are critical. Information retrieval can even be delegated once suitable websites are identified.
- Photocopier is critical. Multiple copies of selected personal documents may be required by one's sponsoring organization. Multiple copies of selected professional documents may be useful with one's peers. Don't assume there will be a good or even functioning printer/copier in the field. For that reason, hardcopies of key reference documents that you bring to the field can be life-saving. Somewhat more elegant is storage in the cloud—making pdfs of selected documents, attaching them in an e-mail, and sending it to yourself.
- Memory sticks (thumb drives) are critical. We take two memory sticks to the field with each laptop. These memory sticks contain core missioncraft information and serve to back-up new disaster work product. We keep a second pair of loaded memory sticks at the field or country office to serve as back-ups in case of field information loss (corrupted sticks, stolen bags, carjacking, evacuation, etc.). Additional memory sticks enable transport of critical information out of the country with departing staff, and serve as gifts for colleagues who face their own information disaster in the field.

Technical Reference Information

The most time-consuming aspect of information management is compiling state-of-the-art technical reference documents. Building this archive is a professional development activity rather than a mission-specific activity. It can be done over time. To facilitate information management, the archive directory structure and file naming conventions should be well-established. Depending on one's aptitudes and interests, the topics may include admin issues, clinical care, disaster plans, human rights, logistics, project management, public health, security, etc. Maintaining the archive requires ongoing work as current documents augment or replace outdated ones. Approximately 15,000 selected reference documents form the core of our archive which is easily transported on an 8 GB memory stick.

An individual mission may yield many new reference documents suitable for archiving. Your sponsoring organization, upon activating you, may provide 1–2 CDs of technical reference information. It's virtually impossible to read all these documents before or during field assignment. When one knows the relevant bibliography, one should not need to. However, it is important to integrate them into an existing electronic archive. One's archive thereby grows in a quantum fashion.

Personal Effects (Document 1.2)

Personal effects are the least challenging domain to prepare. Acquisition long precedes activation—expendables are replaced, degradables are repaired, gear is cleaned and (re)packed. A global "all hazards" approach will simplify commodity selection. One can easily anticipate generic needs in key areas of clothing, toiletries, medication, supplies, and equipment—particularly for tropical and temperate latitudes. Portable adjuncts for exercise and relaxation in activities of daily living contribute to wellness and resilience in the field. While mission-specific climate, culture, and hazard details will ultimately inform personal preparedness for a given disaster, the bulk of personal preparation and packing can be done before disaster strikes.

Unfortunately, packing for field missions is commonly belated and haphazard. Moreover, late packing can hijack the golden opportunity before departure to network and absorb early information emerging from the field.

An indicative personal effects packing list follows in this section. It is not intended to be prescriptive. General comments follow below.

Non-medical Items

- Non-perishable items should be pre-packed. Perishable items, such as batteries or food, can be purchased at the last minute.
- Selected items taken from the pre-packed bags should be identified on a master list so that they can be subsequently restored or replaced.
- Safe water supply is critical. One could never pack enough of it, but do pack 3 portable systems for purification of water from field sources.
- Food is packaged for a day's consumption, and we pack 3 days of it. We tend to conserve it for deep field missions where there is an uncertain food supply. We tend not to use it at country or field offices. However, animal jerky from Australia (kangaroo, crocodile, emu) serves as a useful ice-breaker with visiting dignitaries and local staff.

Medical Items

- Personal medication critical to field function should be transported in hand luggage.
- Selection of other medications and supplies is empirically and epidemiologically based. As emergency and infectious disease physicians, we pack for a broad range of illnesses and injuries which are either common or crescendo (that may prompt untimely evacuation). We do not pack to treat field beneficiaries—they are usually managed thru agency resources in the field. We do pack to treat ourselves and our team members. Although staff health is not the primary job of medical coordinators, individual and team performance, especially in remote locations, can be degraded by easily treatable conditions. Moreover, referential authority and goodwill are important assets that can be markedly enhanced with timely, correct staff medical care. Medication quantities are empirically estimated. These quantities permit drug transport under terms of personal use, yet may serve to treat other members of the team when symptoms are compelling and local referral is not an option.
- Vaccinations should obviously be kept up-to-date. A travel clinic, known to keep stocks of the more unusual vaccines and medications, should be identified at one's home location. It is helpful to be a known patient with local records so that urgent needs may be rapidly addressed.

Survival Supplies

- Survival supplies deserve detailed consideration. In our system, there are 15 different categories of survival supplies (see Document 1.2) which are organized by how they are transported—worn, carried, or stowed. Do not leave this to chance.

Overall, the packing list looks like a lot of stuff for one person. However, in the quantities described above, the list packs into 2 × 22 kg rollaway bags and 2 × 7.5 kg carry on bags. One person in the airport or the field can move them unassisted. Moreover, with the exception of inflammable contents like lighters, all items are transportable under the terms of a commercial aircraft economy ticket.

Document 1.1
PRE-DEPARTURE PREPARATION
Part 1: Information

A. **Geography, Climate, & Weather**

1. Climate and weather data
National Climatic Data Center
http://www.ncdc.noaa.gov/oa/ncdc.html
2. Topographic, aeronautical, and survival maps (1:25,000, gridded, waterproof)
http://www.reliefweb.int/location-maps
http://www.un.org/Depts/Cartographic/english/htmain.htm
http://www.usgs.gov/products/maps/overview
http://www.dmap.co.uk/utmworld.htm
http://earth.google.com/intl/en/index.html
http://www.maps.com/
3. Local maps (1:2500 (1 cm = 25 m) for towns; 1:5000 for villages)
https://www.openstreetmap.org
4. Facilities for medical care, SAR, evacuation

B. **Situation Reports**

ReliefWeb
http://www.reliefweb.int/tools, http://reliefweb.int/briefingkit
GDACS Virtual OSOCC
http://vosocc.unocha.org/
OCHA Humanitarian Response
http://www.humanitarianresponse.info/
WHO Humanitarian Health Action
http://www.who.int/hac/en/
USAID/OFDA Fact Sheets
https://www.usaid.gov/what-we-do/working-crises-and-conflict/responding-times-crisis
Alertnet (global humanitarian news service provided by Reuters Foundation)
http://www.reuters.com/subjects/AlertNet
http://www.reuters.com/subjects/natural-disasters
http://news.trust.org//humanitarian/

C. **Socioeconomic, Consular, & Cultural Reports**

1. Current Comparative World Data
UNDP Development Report
http://hdr.undp.org/en/
2. Country Reports
Country Fact Sheets (Background Notes) (US Dept of State)
http://www.state.gov/r/pa/ei/bgn/
World Factbook (DCI)
https://www.cia.gov/library/publications/the-world-factbook/index.html
International Data and Economic Analysis
https://idea.usaid.gov/
Economist Intelligence Unit
http://www.eiu.com/Default.aspx
ABC-Clio
http://www.abc-clio.com/
World Almanac, Scripps Howard Co
http://www.worldalmanac.com/world-almanac.aspx

3.   Consular and Travel information
  Country Specific Information (US Dept of State)
  https://travel.state.gov/content/studentsabroad/en/beforeyougo/csi.html
  Travel Alerts (US Dept of State)
  https://travel.state.gov/content/passports/en/alertswarnings.html
4.   CultureGrams™
  ProQuest LLC and Brigham Young University
  http://www.culturegrams.com/
5.   Guidebooks
  Lonely Planet

D.   **Health**

1.   Current Comparative World Data
  UNICEF State of the World's Children (SOWC)
  http://www.unicef.org/publications/index_pubs_su.html
  WHO Annual Report
  http://www.who.int/whr/en/index.html
  WHO Country Profiles
  http://www.who.int/countries/en/
  WHO Global Health Observatory Country Data Repository
  http://apps.who.int/ghodata/?theme=country
2.   CDC Travelers Health
  Health Information for International Travel (CDC Yellow Book)
  https://wwwnc.cdc.gov/travel/
  Destination-specific
  https://wwwnc.cdc.gov/travel/destinations/list.htm
  Disease-specific
  https://wwwnc.cdc.gov/travel/page/diseases.htm
3.   Promed
  http://www.promedmail.org/
4.   HealthMap
  http://www.healthmap.org/en/
5.   Control of Communicable Diseases Manual (APHA)
6.   Clinical Guidelines Diagnostic and Treatment Manual (MSF)
7.   Public Health Risk Assessment (WHO)

E.   **Linguistic**

1.   phonetic table
2.   vowel triangle
3.   lexicon template
4.   phrase book (e.g., Language/30 books, Babylon translation software)

F.   **Administrative**

1.   checklists
  pre-deployment checklists
2.   personal documents (copies × 10)
  passport
  tickets
  travel authorization
  country clearance
  International Certificate of Vaccination
  medevac insurance card

photos

driver's license (domestic and international)

pocket medical license

letters of introduction, non-objection

blood type and group

prescriptions for refraction, controlled substances

Note: document distribution

> copy of itinerary in carry-on and checked luggage
>
> copy of personal docs for co-worker traveling with you
>
> copy of personal docs for HR in country office

3. monetary instruments

> cash ($100 s)
>
> credit cards
>
> trinkets

4. designations

> executor
>
> power of attorney
>
> advance directive

5. notifications

> where/how you can be reached
>
> emergency notification contacts and numbers
>
> emergency procedures for family in case of notification

G. Technical References

1. Briefcase/Backpack—hand carried

> memory sticks with missioncraft files
>
> documents (as above)
>
> Logistics & Security file
>
> > country maps
> >
> > Security Briefing Checklist
> >
> > contact list
> >
> > incident command template for listing staff assignments
> >
> > mission plan (hasty planning template)
> >
> > trip plan and vehicle prep
> >
> > comms plan
> >
> > > radio grammar and phonetics
> >
> > security plan
> >
> > > incident report form
> > >
> > > checklists for common hazards—e.g., bomb threat
> > >
> > > 9 line unexploded ordnance form
> > >
> > > 9 line medevac form
> > >
> > > mass casualty incident notification form
> > >
> > > MARCH card
> > >
> > > medevac plan
> > >
> > > contingency plans (abstract)
> > >
> > > evacuation plan (abstract)
> > >
> > > SOPs for ADLs
> >
> > cheat sheets for GPS, HF, satphone
>
> Field Data file
>
> > calendar
> >
> > jurisdictions
> >
> > Layers of Conflict
> >
> > Estimates of Disaster-Affected Population, Damage Estimates

Rapid Epidemiological Assessment
Site Assessment
Sectoral Gap Identification
Health Sector Gap Identification
REA Recommendations
Health Sector Status Summary
cluster lead contacts
security sector Rome Statute definitions (Annex 2)
chlorine concentration table (Annex 3 VI C)
nutrition tables (Annex 3 VII)

Country-Medical file
State of the World's Children (UNICEF)

Country-Political file
country maps
country profile

Misc
water bottle
plastic bottle with electrolyte powder
cell/sat phone
radio handset
pen/pencil sets
waterproof marking pens and isopropyl wipes for maps
color dots for maps
post-its
calculator
leather folio
steno books
plastic bags (folder size)
dummy wallet
poncho
hat
sunglasses

2.   Rollaway/Duffel Bag
Medical Coordination file
Medical Briefing Checklist
Health System Description
Calendar
Jurisdictions
Layers of Conflict
Damage Assessment, Estimates of Disaster-Affected Population
Rapid Epidemiological Assessment
Site Assessment
Feeding Center Assessment
NGO Registration Form
Sectoral Gap Identification
Health Sector Gap Identification
Rapid Epidemiological Assessment Recommendations
Rapid Epidemiological Assessment Annexes
Health Resources Availability Mapping System, Health Services Checklist
Health Sector Status Summary
Health Situation Report
Epidemic Preparedness and Response
Outbreak Investigation Protocol

Outbreak Report in Animals
Medical Coordination Principles of Engagement
Medical Coordination Meeting Agenda, Process
Mission Statement (organization you represent)
Planning Overview
Project Development (WHO)
Priorities Worksheet
Proposal Map
Activity List by Component
Activity List by Public Health Domain (WHO)
Logframe definitions & process
Logframe blank
Project Monitoring & Evaluation Worksheet
Technical Reference Documents (WHO unless noted*)
Rapid Health Assessment Protocols for Emergencies (paperback)
Global Health Cluster Core Indicators
Health Services Checklist
Technical Hazard Sheets
Communicable Diseases Control in Emergencies (paperback)
Surveillance Standards (WHO Early Warning System) (EWAR)
Health Risks for Infectious Diseases
Risk Factors for Outbreak in Emergency Situations
Case Definitions for Health Events
Suggested Alert threshold to Trigger Further Investigation
Steps in Outbreak Management
Outbreak Investigation Protocol
Outbreak Alert Form
Case Investigation Form
Flowchart for Laboratory Confirmation of [list disease]
Diseases Under EWAR Surveillance which Require Laboratory Confirmation
Case for Collection of Specimens in Emergency Conditions
Highlight on Specimen Collection in Emergency Situation
Treatment Guidelines* (from Emergency Health Kit Basic Unit)
Manual for the Health Care of Children in Humanitarian Emergencies
Rationale for Pneumonia Case Detection
Malaria Treatment Guidelines (WHO)
Drugs for Parasitic Infections* (The Medical Letter)
Cholera Outbreak—Assessing the Outbreak Response and Improving Preparedness (paperback)
Epidemic Prep Checklist* (BASICS)
Resources Required for Cholera Treatment Units* (MSF)
Guidelines for Operating Makeshift Treatment Centers in Cholera Epidemics* (ICDDR, B)
Admission History & Physical Sheet* (COTS)
Progress Notes* (COTS)
Guidelines for Measles Surveillance and Outbreak Investigation (WHO & MOH-Ethiopia)
HIV PEP* (CDC)
Drugs for HIV Infection* (Medical Letter)
Weekly Morbidity form (daily entries to arrive at weekly totals)
Weekly Mortality form (daily entries to arrive at weekly totals)
Weekly Surveillance Reporting Form M&M (weekly totals only)
Surveillance System Data Flow Chart*
List of WHO Guidelines of Communicable Diseases (In: CD Profiles for [list country])
Public Health Emergency Guidelines

Kit Descriptions (list)

Interagency Emergency Health Kit (paperback)

Trauma Diseases Kits (list)

Emergency Library Kit (list)

WHO Handbook for Emergency Field Operations or Managing WHO Humanitarian Response
      in the Field

Actions in a Level 3 Emergency

Sample Humanitarian Program Cycle calendar

WHO Performance Standards (ERF)

Effects and Response Priorities in Different Types of Emergencies

Health Sector Response Strategy

Contingency Plan Template for the Health Sector

Health Cluster Performance Assessment and Monitoring Tool Partner Form

WHO's Core Functions

WHO Gender Mainstreaming

Health in the Sustainable Development Goals*

ICDDR

COTS Program CD with job action cards

Misc References

Concentrations of Cl Solutions for Disinfection

Materials Required for House (Construction)

Guidelines for Maintaining and Managing the Vaccine Cold Chain (CDC)

Outline Strategy for Malaria Control (WHO\RBM planning template)

Red Cross Wound Classification

OFDA

Field Operations Guide

WMD

MARCH card × 2

CDC blast card × 2

Chemical agent profiles

Biological agent profiles

How to Handle Anthrax and Other Biological Agent Threats (CDC)

Document 1.2
PRE-DEPARTURE PREPARATION
Part 2: Personal Effects

A.   **Clothing**

B.   **Toiletries**

C.   **Activities of Daily Living**

D.   **Medications**

    1.   Analgesics
    2.   Anaphylaxis/atopy
    3.   Antibiotics
    4.   Antiparasitics
    5.   Antivirals
    6.   Cardiac
    7.   Dental
    8.   Dermatologics
    9.   ENT
    10.   Gastrointestinal
    11.   Gyn
    12.   Psychiatric
    13.   Miscellaneous

E.   **Medical Supplies**

    1.   Wound Care
    2.   General Medical

F.   **Survival Supplies**

    1.   Currency & Documentation
    2.   Communication
    3.   Site
    4.   Safety
    5.   Security
    6.   Water
    7.   Sanitation
    8.   Food
    9.   Clothing
    10.   Shelter
    11.   Vector Control
    12.   Mechanical Advantage
    13.   Drugs, Supplies, & First Aid
    14.   Relaxation Aids
    15.   Gifts
    16.   Emergency Evacuation

G.   **Sequence**

    1.   Mental
    2.   Physical
    3.   Medical
    4.   Administrative

A.   **Clothing**

hat × 2 (e.g., Ultimate Hat®, Tampa, FL, USA)

bandana (muslin triangular bandage)—12 uses: sun hat, head scarf, evaporation collar, dust mask, water filter, tourni-
   quet, wound dressing, wound bandage, extremity splint ties, sling, restraints, tinder for fire

vest

poncho

poncho liner

waterproof outer shell

polar fleece

thermal underwear

gloves

gortex suit

long pants, long sleeve shirts, short sleeve shirts × 3

short pants, t-shirt × 2

circle scarf

belts × 2

underwear × 4

hiking boots,

boot laces × 3

hiking socks (wool) × 4

liner socks (silk, polypro) × 4

running shoes

sandals, flip-flops, or sand shoes (e.g., Crocs™, Boulder, CO, USA)

bathing suit

scrub suit

work gloves

B.   **Toiletries**

hand towel
washing vessel
soap (bar, shampoo, detergent)
wash sponge
nail brush
hand sanitizer
disposable wipes (e.g., Wash 'N Dri®, Clorox Co, Oakland, CA, USA)
reusable wipes (e.g., Handi-Wipes®, Clorox Co, Oakland, CA, USA)
toilet paper in plastic bag
cotton swabs
toothbrush, toothpaste, floss
nail clippers, file
comb
pocket mirror
scissors, tweezers
razor, shave cream
sanitary pads, tampons
condoms, diaphragms

C.   **Activities of Daily Living** (utility, versatility, simplicity, portability, durability, availability, low cost)

flashlight (LED) (e.g., SureFire®, Fountain Valley, CA, USA), filters, lanyard
headlight (LED)
strobe light
lighter
candles, matches (waterproof)
knife, scissors
can opener, bottle opener
utility tool (e.g., Leatherman®, Portland, OR, USA)
pen, pencil
paper (notepads, steno pads, quadrille pads)
eyeglasses (sunglasses, reading glasses, protective glasses)
eyeglasses repair kit
lens solution, tissues (glasses and camera)
earplugs, eyeshades
duct tape
nylon cord
cable ties
safety pins, paper clips, rubber bands
sewing kit
glue (paper, synthetics)
combination lock (padlock, chain lock, combilock)
containers
            bumbag
            daypack
            rollaway bag
            waterproof liner, waterproof bag cover
            stuff sacks
            food/ORS/soap containers (e.g., Nalgene®, Rochester, NY, USA)
            plastic bags (quart, gallon, 4 gallon, 8 gallon, 40 gallon)
            zip lock bags, twist ties
            plastic sleeves for posted notices
            pill bottles for meds and food spices
            collapsible bag for overnight or emergency evacuation
door lock, door jam (1″ screw)
steel wool (useful for batteries, stripped screws), wire
tape measure
thermometer (outdoor)
watch
alarm clock
batteries (AA, AAA, C, camera, 123A 3-volt Lithium)
USB car charger
portable solar battery charger (e.g., Goal Zero)
business cards
agency/office decals
red stamp with company name
manila folders

cameras
calculators
voice recorder
music player (mp3)
short wave radio
laptop computer, tablet, battery, laptop charger (e.g., Zolt), surge protector, locking cable
wallet, dummy wallet, money belt
paperback book
dice, cards
gifts (lapel pins, commemorative coins, utility tools)

D. **Medications**

    1. Analgesics

Aspirin	325 mg tabs
Acetaminophen (APAP)	325 mg tabs
APAP + Codeine	300/30 mg tabs
Oxycodone	5 mg tabs
Morphine sulfate	injection, buccal
Fentanyl	50 µg/h patch

    2. Anaphylaxis/atopy

Epinephrine	1:1000 injection
Diphenhydramine	50 mg tabs, injection
Prednisone	20 mg tabs
Albuterol, Salbutamol	metered-dose inhaler

    3. Antibiotics

Dicloxacillin	500 mg tabs
Cephalexin	500 mg tabs
Azithromycin	500 mg tabs
Doxycycline	100 mg tabs
Ciprofloxacin	500 mg tabs
Trimethoprim + Sulfa	400 mg/80 mg tabs
Metronidazole	500 mg tabs
Ceftriaxone	injection

    4. Antiparasitics

Artemether + Lumefantrine	20 mg/120 mg = Coartem
	1 mg/kg Artemether PO/PR at 0, 8, 24, 36, 48, 60 h
	adults 4 tabs/dose; < 1 yr. not recommended
Mefloquine	250 mg tabs
Chloroquine	500 mg tabs
Quinine sulfate	325 mg tabs
Lindane 1% lotion, shampoo	
Mebendazole	100 mg tabs
Tinidazole	500 mg tabs

    5. Antivirals

Oseltamivir	75 mg caps
Acyclovir	200 mg caps
Zidovudine (AZT) + Lamivudine (3TC)	300 mg/150 mg = Combivir (1 BID)
Lopinavir (LPV) + Ritonavir (RTV)	400 mg/100 mg = Kaletra (1 BID or 2 QD)
Combivir + Kaletra	indicated for PEP

    6. Cardiac

Enoxaparin	40 or 80 mg pre-filled syringes
Furosemide	20 mg injection
Nitroglycerin	0.4 mg tabs, pump spray

7. Dental

   Carbamide peroxide   10% oral solution
   Temporary bond

8. Dermatologics

   sunscreen (SPF 30+)
   lip balm/sunscreen
   talc
   Zinc undecylenate   20% powder
   Miconazole   2% cream, 200 mg vaginal tabs
   Betamethasone   0.1% cream
   Silver sulfadiazine   1% cream

9. ENT/Ophtho

   Chlorpheniramine   4 mg tabs
   Pseudoephedrine   60 mg tabs
   Cortisporin   otic suspension
   Tetrahydrozoline   0.05% solution
   Proparacaine   0.5% solution
   Erythromycin   5% ophthalmic ointment
   Sulfacetamide   10% ophthalmic solution

10. GI

    Loperamide   2 mg caps
    Bismuth subsalicylate   tabs
    Ondansetron   4 mg wafers
    Prochlorperazine   25 mg suppository, injection
    Scopolamine   dermal patches

11. Gyn

    Ethinylestradiol + Levonorgestrel   0.05 mg/0.25 mg

12. Psyc

    Triazolam   0.25 mg tabs
    Temazepam   10 mg tabs
    Diazepam   10 mg tabs, injection
    Droperidol   injection
    Haloperidol   5 mg tabs, injection
    Benztropine   2 mg injection

13. Misc

    Acetazolamide   250 mg tabs
    Multi-vits

NB   Many countries require documentation for restricted medications taken through customs.

E. **Medical Supplies**

   1.   Wound Care

       bandaids
       moleskin, molefoam
       transparent dressings (e.g., Tegaderm™, 3 M, St. Paul, MN, USA)
       blister pads (e.g., Spenco® 2nd Skin®, Spenco Medical Corp, Waco, TX, USA)
       alcohol swabs
       povidone-iodine swabs, solution
       scrub brushes (antiseptic impregnated)
       lidocaine 2% injection
       syringes (injection, irrigation)
       needles
       irrigation cannulas
       splinter forceps
       scalpel
       tissue adhesive (e.g., n-Butyl cyanoacrylate)
       needle holder
       suture
       tissue scissors
       penrose drain
       butterflies
       antibiotic ointment
       impregnated, non-adherent dressings
       sponges (menstrual pads for copious discharge)
       bandages (crepe, gauze, elastic)
       adhesive tape
       bandage scissors
       cravats
       nylon straps, velcro closures
       ensolite splints (e.g., SAM® splints, Wilsonville, OR, USA)
       individual first aid kit (in areas of high velocity or explosive munitions)
          tourniquet, gauze, trauma bandage, nasopharyngeal airway, occlusive dressing, trauma shears, latex gloves, trauma card, marker

   2.   General Medical

       sphygmomanometer (aneroid)
       stethoscope c spare earpieces
       thermometer (PO, PR)
       malaria RDT (e.g., Paracheck-Pf®, Orchid Biomedical Systems, Goa, India)
       otoscope, ophthalmoscope
       gloves (latex, sterile and non-sterile)
       masks (with vial of oil-based volatile perfume as needed for death investigations)
       tongue blades
       dental kit with temporary restoration
       tracheostomy tube
       IV catheters
       heparin lock
       sterile water for injection
       foley catheter
       sterile lubricant

F. **Survival Supplies**

1. Currency and Documentation

    cash[+], dummy wallet[+]
    passport[+] (always keep with you in deep field)
    medevac card[+]
    copy of your organization's mission statement

2. Communication

    cell phone[+]
    sat phone[++] (e.g., Thuraya SatSleeve, Thuraya dual-mode phone)
    wireless battery case[+] (e.g., Mophie®), car charger
    radio[++] (VHF—veld areas; UHF—urban areas)
    contact info[+]
    point & talk cards[+]
    pen/pencil[+]
    pad of paper[+]
    language reference[+] (e.g., Language/30 books, Educational Services Corp, Folly Beach, SC, USA)
    flashlight[+,#] with lanyard and red filter
    headlight[+,#]
    strobe light[#]
    batteries[+,#]
    portable battery charger (with USB ports)[+]
    solar charger[#]
    lighter[+]
    whistle[+] (plastic body, cork ball) with lanyard
    signaling mirror with focusing screen[+]
    surveyor's tape
    personal tracker locator[#]
    personal locator beacon[#]

3. Site

    compass[+] (military lensatic)
    maps[++] (1:25,000)
    GPS[++] (e.g., Garmin®, Olathe, KS, USA)

4. Safety

    dust mask[+] (N 95)
    smoke hood

5. Security

    utility tool[+]
    cable ties[+]
    alarm

6. Water

    cup[+]
    water bottle[++] (1.5 L)
    solute bottle[++] (0.5 L)
    water purification tablets[+] (e.g., Potable Aqua®, Jackson, WI, USA)
    water purification straw[+] (7 micron micropore filter)

mesh strainer[+] (coffee filter)
electrolytes & flavorings[+, ++] (e.g., sports drinks, tea, coffee, cocoa, bouillon)
water bladder (collapsible)
plastic tubing (2′)
funnel (conical or small plastic bag)
filtration pump[##] (e.g., Katadyn water filters, Wallisellen-Zurich, Switzerland)
bottled water[##]

7.   Sanitation

toilet paper[+, #]
disposable wipes[+, #]
reusable wipes[+]
soap bar[+, #]
shampoo[#]
sponge[#]
comb[#]
toothbrush, toothpaste[#]

8.   Food

gorp[++] (dried fruit, dried meat, trail mix, granola bars, hard candy)
food[##] (meals, ready-to-eat or 1-day bags)
       breakfast—packet oatmeal, packet soup
       lunch— animal jerky (beef, kangaroo, emu, crocodile), dried fruits, spreads (peanut butter, chutney),
       dinner—freeze-dried/packet meals (soup, pasta, couscous, rice, mixed veg)
spices
utensils[+]
camp cup, pie pan
plastic squeeze tubes, containers
aluminum foil

9.   Clothing

hiking boots[*]
extra laces[+]
hiking socks[*, #]
liner socks[*, +, #]
long pants[*]
long sleeve shirt[*]
vest[*]
bandana/triangular bandage[+]
hat[*]
poncho[++]
flip-flops or sand shoes[#]
bathing suit[#]
hand towel[#] (quick drying)
scrub suit[#]

10.   Shelter

poncho[++] (as above)
space blanket[#] (gold reflective)
550 paracord[#]
duct tape[#]
sleeping bag with waterproof cover[#] (3 season)

sleeping sheet# (silk)
air pillow#
ground pad## (ensolite, polyurethane)
air mattress## (e.g., Therm-a-Rest®, Cascade Designs, Seattle, WA, USA), repair kit
tent, poles, pegs
lighter, fire starter# (eg Lightning-Strike™, magnesium bar), waterproof matches#, tinder# (eg Tinder-Quik, cotton balls, petroleum jelly)
spade##

11. Vector Control

DEET repellent+, # (30–50%)
insecticide treated bednet (ITN) with 6 × 2 m lanyards#
pyrethrum insecticide (for pants legs and shirt sleeves)
permethrin 2% emulsifiable concentrate (for clothes and ITN diluted 1:3 with water)
sweat bands (head, extremities) for repellent impregnation

12. Mechanical Advantage

rope## (5/8″ kernmantle) × 50′
tube webbing## (1″ nylon) × 2 m
carabiners## (10 cm, aluminum, locking) × 2
figure-of-8## (aluminum c ears)
pulleys## (2″ aluminum)
hammock

13. Drugs, Supplies, & First Aid

sunscreen+
lip balm+
talc#
ciprofloxacin+
loperamide+
triazolam#
bandaids+, #
moleskin#
antibiotic ointment+
latex gloves+
earplugs#
eyeshades#
individual first aid kit#

14. Relaxation Aids

paperback book
music player# (mp3)
playing cards, dice

15. Gifts

lapel pins+
cigarettes+
utility tools+
cameras

16. Emergency Evacuation (Personal Survival Kit comprises selections from groups 1-15)

     *   dress it—hiking boots, hiking socks, liner socks, long pants, long sleeve shirt, vest, hat

     +   carry it (bumbag)—cash, dummy wallet, passport, medevac card, cell phone, wireless battery case, contact info, blood-chit, point & talk cards, language reference, flashlight, headlight, batteries, portable battery charger (with USB ports), lighter, whistle, signaling mirror, compass, dust mask, utility tool, cable ties, cup, purification tablets, purification straw, mesh strainer, electrolytes in sachets, toilet paper, disposable wipes, reusable wipes, soap bar, utensils, extra laces, liner socks, bandana, DEET, sunscreen, lip balm, ciprofloxacin, loperamide, latex gloves, work gloves, lapel pins, cigarettes; (outer pocket) pen/pencil, pad of paper, bandaids, antibiotic ointment

     ++   carry it (briefcase bag/handbag)— sat phone, radio, maps, GPS, full water bottle, solute bottle, electrolytes, gorp, poncho

     #   stow it (backpack—8 subpacks)

         comms pack (solar charger, strobe light, personal tracker locator, personal locator beacon)

         personal protection pack (poncho, space blanket, 550 paracord, duct tape, fire starter, waterproof matches, tinder)

         toiletry pack (toilet paper, disposable wipes, soap bar, shampoo, sponge, comb, toothbrush, toothpaste)

         foot pack (hiking socks, liner socks, extra laces, talc, bandaids, moleskin)

         bathing pack (flip flops, bathing suit, hand towel)

         ITN pack (ITN, DEET, 6 × 2m lanyards)

         sleeping pack (sleeping bag with cover, sleeping sheet, space blanket, scrub suit, air pillow, flashlight, headlight, batteries, earplugs, eyeshades, mp3 player, triazolam)

         individual first aid kit

     ##   stow it (trunk of 4 × 4)—filtration pump, water bladder, bottled water, MREs, ground pad, air mattress, spade, rope, tube webbing, carabiners, figure-of-8, pulleys

G.   Sequence

1. Mental

   preparedness >
   briefing

2. Physical

   conditioning >
   bioadaption

3. Medical

   DPT, OPV, MMR, HA, HB, influenza, meningococcus, rabies, cholera, YF, JE >
   oral typhoid >
   malaria >
   GI

4. Administrative

   medical clearance, vaccination >
   staff health and medevac >
   visas, tickets, travel insurance >
   field safety and security >
   in-country accommodation and transportation

Contents

Guidance Notes

Briefing is one of the weakest parts of professional practice in the disaster health sector. Headquarters and regional offices often lack detailed knowledge about the field and commonly refer incoming health personnel with specific questions to the field. Once in the field, health personnel may find their predecessors have already left. When overlap does occur, briefings in the acute disaster setting may be rushed and ad hoc. Standardized information checklists, routine tools in aviation safety and emerging tools in patient safety, are rarely used. Thus, just as shift change can harm patients in emergency departments and hospital wards, so can shift change harm beneficiaries in disaster health programs. You should not ratify malpractice by tolerating a poor briefing, and you should certainly not propagate it on your successor. Ultimately, a bad handover is the bane of the receiver. Once the incumbent leaves the field, the successor owns the problem whether he knows about it or not. So, whether you are first in the field, or next to last, briefing is a leadership opportunity to bring order to chaos.

Security Checklist (Document 2.1)

Security briefing is relatively straightforward. The key points for the health officer are:

- Hold your sponsoring agency fully accountable for a comprehensive safety and security plan.
- Ask for detailed sub-plans—communications plan, medevac plan, hazard-specific contingency plans, and team evacuation plan. While such plans may not exist, particularly early in disaster, you must be prepared to contribute to their development.

A field health officer has a compliance role in a communications plan, a lead role in a medevac plan, a supportive role in a hazard-specific contingency plan, and an unpredictable role in a team evacuation plan.

• Know the SOPs, follow them, and ensure your team knows them. Non-compliance with security procedures is cause for summary dismissal from the field.

Medical Handover Checklist (Document 2.2)

Medical briefing is core content for the medical coordinator. There is a lot of information here. You will not get it all in your field briefing, and perhaps not in your first week on the job. Indeed, you can be overbearing if you pursue it too compulsively. Nonetheless, it's important to clearly envision the information building blocks of competent medical coordination. Many of the reference documents do not need to be written by ex-pat staff. They merely need to be sourced. With conceptual clarity and due diligence, the complete reference list should emerge over time.

It is unconscionable for the medical coordinator, especially one who has worked for months in the field, to content himself with readily available information (Document 2.2 A, B, F, G) at the expense of elusive information which is most relevant to the beneficiaries (Document 2.2 C, D, H). Important examples are the health system profile (Document 2.2 C2) and the emergency management system profile (Document 2.2 C4). These profiles remain a rarity among country-specific descriptions commonly found on websites of UN and donor aid agencies. For example, WHO posts country health profiles on the website of its country offices. However, their structure is variable, their contents typically relate to health development, and their data are typically stale. In general, detailed health system and emergency management system profiles are difficult to source out-of-country and need to be compiled in-country. While operational tempo in disaster relief does not lend itself to detailed systems' analysis, familiarity with these systems remains mission critical. For this reason, outline profiles for these systems are presented as the first two tools (Tools 2.T1 and 2.T2) in the section. The other tools of the section are self-explanatory.

Document 2.1
SECURITY CHECKLIST

Safety & Security Officer

Name

Contact details

Emergency services phone #s

Safety and Security Plan (SSP)

Plan	Received (Y/N)	Obtain From
SSP comprehensive		
Comms Plan		
Medevac Plan		
Contingency Plans		
Evacuation Plan		
SOPs	**Received (Y/N)**	**Obtain From**
Security update		
Activities of Daily Living		
Comms (primary, alternate, contingency, & emergency)		
Travel (primary, alternate, contingency, & emergency)		
Routine check-in/notifications		

Current Situation **ETHANE**	**Tactical Situation** **METT-T**	**Operations Orders** **SMEAC**
Exact location (of incident)	Mission	Situation
Type of incident (hazard)	Enemy	Mission
Hazards present	Terrain	Execution
Access for emergency vehicles	Troops	Admin & logistics
Number & severity of casualties	Time available	Command & signals
Emergency services present & needed		

Document 2.1
ORIENTATION TO THE OFFICE

Find building entry/exit points.

Find landlines and sat phones.

Find smoke detectors, fire alarms, and fire extinguishers.

Find smoke hoods, hard hats, and flashlights.

Find first aid kit.

Find protected room for shelter-in-place. Otherwise, find toilet block (often structurally sounder than main building with ventilation and water source).

Find building escape route and outside rally point.

Find escape routes from the neighborhood.

Get GPS coordinates for office and home. Know 3 routes between them.

Know how to call the security officer, neighborhood warder, team leader, and phone tree contacts.

Document 2.2
MEDICAL HANDOVER CHECKLIST

A. **Scope of Work/Terms of Reference**

1. Responsibilities
   a. key deliverables
2. Authorities (#1 and #2 must be compatible)
   a. staff
   b. material (comms, vehicles)
   c. financial (accounts, cash)
3. Reporting requirements—to whom, how often, what level of detail

B. **Agency Background and Work Environment**

1. Mission statement and host country permission to operate
2. Organogram
3. Contact lists
4. Administrative rules
   a. staff support (secretarial, logistics)
   b. key policies (e.g., security, resource management, media)
   c. travel authorization & security clearance
   d. length of assignment
   e. work week, pay schedule
   f. benefits—insurance, liability limits
5. Security plan, security briefing
   a. security officer address, contact details
   b. warden address, contact details
6. Communications plan, comms briefing
   a. radio room location, contact details
7. Medical evacuation plan, health briefing
   a. medical facility location, contact details
8. Work processes and products
   a. correspondence
      (1) e-mail address
      (2) list serves
   b. reporting
      (1) sitreps (monthly)
      (2) cluster bulletins (monthly)
      (3) EWARN reports (weekly)
      (4) epidemic-specific reports (ad hoc)
      (5) maps
   c. archives
      (1) shared drives
      (2) google docs (invitation)
9. Office address, contact details
10. Home address, contact details

C. **Host Country Government and Health System**

1. Country profile (e.g., DCI factbook)
2. Health system profile
3. Public health profile (e.g., WHO Communicable Disease Profile)
4. Emergency management system profile
5. MOH organogram
6. Current government appeals
7. Status of relationships

D. **Beneficiaries**

1. Local map (1:100,000)
2. Local map with camp locations
3. Table of # refugees and # HoH by (sub)districts
4. Table of # refugee sites by (sub)districts and site population size bracket (<5000, 5000–10,000, 10,000–15,000 etc.)
5. Table of # refugee sites and # refugees by health center catchments
6. Quantitation of vulnerable groups—U5, orphaned, pregnant, etc.
7. Status of relationships

E. **Incident Management**

1. Organogram
2. Job action sheets, position task books
3. Local (country) office repurposing plan
4. Staff succession plan and absences from key positions
5. Incident action plan
6. Delegated authorities (finance)
7. Upcoming deliverables in humanitarian program cycle and emergency response framework

F. **Cluster Process**

1. Partners and key contacts
2. 4 Ws (who-what-where-when or area-activity matrix)
3. HeRAMS
4. Gap analysis—qualitative assessment of unmet need
5. Integrated subsector planning (pairing of iNGOs with local NGOs and health structures)
6. Strategic response plan
7. Multi-party (added value) actions in hazard mitigation, vulnerability reduction
8. Status of relationships

G. **Project Management**

1. Project plans of action
2. Periodic progress reports—copies (hard and soft) of last 3 monthly medical reports with instructions on locating original source documents from which the reports were compiled
3. Other work product
   a. assessments
   b. appeals
   c. evaluations
   d. prevention-preparedness-mitigation-response plans
4. Human resources documents
   a. project organogram
   b. weekly schedule of internal and external meetings to attend
   c. future staff needs
5. Material resources documents
   a. logistics assets and allocation
   b. current shortages in critical goods
   c. inventory of warehoused commodities
6. Financial resources documents
   a. donor alert
   b. flash appeal
   c. regional office funds available
   d. headquarters funds available

7. Key documentation—existing contracts, mous, correspondence
8. List of issues which will need attention or explode within the first week on the job—and analysis of those issues
9. List of correspondence which will need reply within the first week on the job
10. Health sector status summary
11. Assessment of current problems in non-clinical sectors which impact medical care
    a. security
    b. logistics
    c. environmental health—water, food, sanitation, shelter, vector control
    d. preventive medicine—labs to confirm index cases of epidemics, vaccine stocks

H.   **Normative Technical Practices**

1. Standardized case management
   a. clinical case definitions
   b. treatment protocols authorized by MOH in host country
   c. other clinical protocols (standard precautions, injection safety, medical waste mgmt)
   d. essential drugs and rational drug use
   e. secondary prevention
   f. referral guidelines
2. Epidemiological surveillance
   a. clinical case definitions
   b. site recording sheets
   c. weekly surveillance report forms
   d. analysis and reporting process—description and diagram
   e. responsible official
   f. recent field studies
3. Epidemic preparedness
   a. list of disease outbreaks and epidemic threats
   b. plan of action
   c. clinical case definitions (especially if differ from surveillance definition)
   d. case management guidelines for communicable diseases with epidemic potential
   e. outbreak management protocol
   f. secondary prevention
   g. resource prepositioning and stockpiles
   h. information management
   i. contingency planning
4. Other

I.   **Meetings Schedule**

1. Local agency
2. Health cluster
3. Inter-cluster working group
4. Regional office and headquarters teleconferences

J.   **Contact List** (office address, phone, and contact list)

1. Index organization
2. Government officials
3. UN, IOs
4. NGOs
5. Focal points for document distribution

Tool 2.T1
HEALTH SYSTEM PROFILE

I.   CONTEXT

    A.   **Legal Framework**

    B.   **Rights Framework** (to health care)

    C.   **Social Participation and Control**

II.   POLITICAL JURISDICTIONS

III.   INDICATORS

    A.   **Access to Essential Services** (see UNICEF [1], WHO [2] for country data)

        1.   Public utilities (infrastructure)
            a.   % with improved water
            b.   % with improved sanitation
            c.   % with electricity
            d.   % with telephones/television
        2.   Health services
            a.   skilled health care workers (all)/10,000 p   (23)
            b.   physicians/10,000 p   (0.2)
            c.   nurses/10,000 p   (1)
            d.   midwives/10,000 p   (1)
            e.   community health workers/10,000 p   (10)
            f.   % population with provider coverage   (100%)
            g.   consultations/p/yr   (1)
            h.   % pregnancies receiving antenatal care   (100%)
            i.   % deliveries attended by trained staff   (90%)
            j.   % immunization rates—measles vac in 1 y/o   (90%)
            k.   hospital beds/10,000 p   (10)
            l.   health facilities with BEOC, CEOC/500,000 p   (4, 1)
            m.   admissions/10,000 p
        3.   Underserved areas (by location and type of service)

    B.   **Health Status** (see UNICEF [1], WHO [2] for country data)

        1.   Mortality and other rates
            a.   CBR   (10–50)
            b.   CMR   (5–25)
            c.   AGR   (%)
            d.   IMR   (3–200)
            e.   U5MR   (3–300)
            f.   MMR   (5–2100)
            g. E_0 at birth M/F/T   (40–85)
            h.   TFR   (2–8)
        2.   Nutritional status
            a.   caloric intake/p/d (2100 kcal)
            b.   % infants with low birth weight (LBW) (7% with <2.5 kg)
            c.   % U5 with growth faltering (30%)

        d. % U5 with global acute malnutrition (GAM) (10%)

        e. % with micronutrient deficiencies (vitamins A–D; Fe, I)

        f. % of food supply from international food assistance (WFP, NGOs)

  3. Endemic diseases

        a. HIV prevalence

        b. TB prevalence

        c. malaria incidence

        d. other major diseases

  4. Health beliefs and traditions

  5. Sources of care

  6. Referral system

IV. SYSTEM DESCRIPTION

A. Public Health Services

  1. Disease prevention

        a. primary prevention

           (1) vaccine coverage rates for major antigens (EPI coverage rate > 90%)

                (a) measles

                (b) DPT

           (2) vaccine stocks   quantity available   location

                (a) measles

                (b) DPT

                (c) polio

                (d) hepatitis B

                (e) other

           (3) cold chain adequacy

           (4) staff adequacy

           (5) transport adequacy

           (6) most recent campaign in area

                (a) location

                (b) dates

                (c) organizer

                (d) coverage

           (7) other VPIs of epidemic potential

        b. communicable disease control programs   Y/N   issues

           (1) diarrhea

           (2) ARI

           (3) malaria

           (4) HIV

           (5) TB

           (6) other

  2. Epidemiological surveillance system (CDC [3])

        a. system objectives

           (1) case detection (CDs, NCDs e.g., malnutrition)

           (2) outbreak detection

           (3) epidemic forecasting

           (4) trend monitoring

           (5) priority setting

           (6) workload estimation

           (7) resource targeting & health program activity

           (8) intervention evaluation

    b.   health events/indicator conditions and case definitions

    c.   system components and flow chart of operations
- (1) what is the population under surveillance?
- (2) what is the time period of data collection?
- (3) what data are collected (standardized forms)?
- (4) who provides the data?
- (5) how are data transmitted?
- (6) how are data stored?
- (7) who analyzes the data?
- (8) how are data analyzed and how often?
- (9) how often are reports generated?
- (10) to whom are reports disseminated?
- (11) how are reports disseminated?

    d.   level of usefulness (users of data and actions taken)

    e.   system attributes
- (1) simplicity
- (2) flexibility
- (3) sensitivity
- (4) reliability
- (5) acceptability
- (6) positive predictive value
- (7) representativeness
- (8) timeliness

    f.   system resource requirements (direct costs)
- (1) personnel
- (2) other (computer & office equipment, travel, training, mobile phone)

3.   Epidemic preparedness and outbreak response

    a.   plan of action and coordinating committee
- (1) public health incident command system (PHICS)
- (2) cholera command and control center (C4)

    b.   clinical case definitions

    c.   case mgmt guidelines for communicable diseases with epidemic potential

    d.   outbreak mgmt protocol
- (1) surveillance definitions
- (2) alert thresholds
- (3) rapid response teams to investigate case reports
- (4) epidemic investigation kits to use
- (5) specimens to collect
- (6) labs to verify diagnosis (including sample sharing for confirmatory testing)
- (7) patients to identify, isolate, and treat (inpatient and outpatient settings)
  - (a) isolation areas to organize
  - (b) treatments to plan
- (8) contacts to trace and ? quarantine
- (9) hotlines to use for notifiable diseases and investigation of rumor

    e.   primary and secondary prevention
- (1) infection control protocols
- (2) commodities
  - (a) vaccines (e.g., measles, meningitis)
  - (b) drugs (e.g., prophylactic meds)
  - (c) chemicals (e.g., soap, Ca hypochlorite)
  - (d) supplies (e.g., chlorimetric and colimetric monitors)
  - (e) equipment (e.g., PPE)

    f.   resource prepositioning (stockpiles, supply chain)

    g.   information mgmt and crisis communication (media strategy)

          (1)   health authorities, WHO
          (2)   political authorities
          (3)   community leaders and public
              (a)   social mobilization
              (b)   hygiene promotion and health education
              (c)   behavioral change communication (BCC)
    h.   contingency planning for epidemic consequences
          (1)   provision of essential services (lifelines)
          (2)   corpse mgmt
 4.   Health promotion
    a.   targeted diseases
          (1)   acute epidemic diseases
          (2)   chronic diseases—HTN, DM, HIV/TB, asthma
    b.   health promotion activities
          (1)   community health education
          (2)   provider education
 5.   Health protection (if significant to disaster response)
    a.   air quality (e.g., wildfires, volcanic eruptions)
    b.   injury control
    c.   occupational health and safety
    d.   hazardous materials (e.g., chemical releases)
    e.   disaster risk reduction (e.g., safe hospitals)
 6.   Issues summary

B.   **Health Facilities and Clinical Services**

		Mobile Clinics	Fixed Clinics	Health Centers	District Hospitals
1.	Quantity				
2.	Catchment population				
	benchmark		5–10 k	<50 k	100 k
3.	Access to facility				
	benchmark		self	self	referral
4.	Staffing				
	a. quantity (~1/1000 population)				
	benchmark		2–5	5–10	variable
	b. skill mix				
	benchmark		1 HCW	5 HCW, 1 MD	MD, 1 surg
5.	Caseload (1–10% of catchment population/d)				
	benchmark		1%	1%	
6.	Bed capacity (10/10,000 population)				
7.	Bed occupancy				
8.	Referral load (10% of caseload)				
	benchmark		10%	10%	
9.	Referral system				
10.	Clinical services	OPD, ORS	→ + IPD, L&D		→ + OR
	a. departments/units (verify functioning of expected services)				
	(1) clinical				
	(a) OPD		+	+	+
	(b) IPD		-	+	+
	(c) L&D		-	+	+
	(d) surgery		-	+/-	+
	(e) other				
	(2) dispensary		+/-	+	+
	(3) diagnostic lab		+/-	+	+
	(4) blood bank		-	-	+
	(5) radiology		-	-	+

b. special services (verify quality of care)
   (1) child health
      (a) EPI
      (b) IMCI
      (c) child protection
   (2) reproductive health (20% of P_T are F 15–44 yr; 20% (4% of P_T) are pregnant, 20% (4% of P_T) are lactating)
      (a) identify RH lead agency
      (b) prevent and manage consequences of sexual & gender-based violence (SGBV)
         (i) emergency contraception (post rape)
      (c) reduce HIV transmission
         (i) abstain, be faithful, use condoms (ABCs)
         (ii) standard precautions
         (iii) treatment of STIs
         (iv) PMTCT
      (d) safe motherhood—basic & comprehensive emergency OB care
         (i) antenatal care
         (ii) professional midwifery
         (iii) clean delivery
         (iv) essential newborn care
         (v) referral options
      (e) family planning
         (i) general contraception
   (3) trauma
      (a) (para)military conflict
      (b) domestic violence
      (c) rape
      (d) motor vehicle trauma
   (4) mental health
      (a) adjustment disorders (e.g., debilitating grief reactions)
      (b) psychiatric disease (e.g., psychoses, affective disorders) (severe—baseline 2–3% of P_T + 1% increase post-disaster (net 50% increase); mild-mod—baseline 10% of P_T + 5–10% increase post-disaster (net 50–100% increase))
      (c) violence
      (d) drug abuse
   (5) chronic diseases (20% of P_T)
      (a) HTN
      (b) DM
      (c) HIV/TB
      (d) asthma
      (e) other
c. standardized case management
   (1) clinical case definitions
   (2) treatment protocols (ORS + Zn, ABX, ACT, IPT, and ITN will save 75% of U5 deaths)
   (3) other clinical protocols (standard precautions, injection safety, medical waste mgmt)
   (4) essential (standard) drugs and rational drug use
      (a) EHKs
      (b) specialty kits
   (5) referral guidelines
   (6) secondary prevention
d. infection control
   (1) dedicated staff
   (2) hand washing facilities

        (3)   stocks of essential supplies (soap, gloves, masks, gowns)

        (4)   infection control protocols

        (5)   compliance

11. Utilities

    a. power supply

    b. water supply

    c. excreta disposal/septic system

12. Issues summary

C. Human Resources

	Available/10,000 p	Needed (quantity)

1. Basic (not vocationally trained)

    a. traditional birth attendant

    b. community health worker

    c. nurse's aide

    d. other applicable

2. Mid, High (vocationally trained)

    a. surgical/lab/pharmacy tech

    b. nurse

    c. midwife

    d. pharmacist

    e. doctor

    f. health facility administrator

    g. public health staff (identify)

    h. other applicable

3. Major areas with staff shortage

4. Reasons for staff shortage (e.g., security, migration, salary)

5. Issues summary

D. Essential Medical Products and Technologies

1. National standards

    a. essential medicines formulary

    b. standardized equipment per level of care

    c. diagnostic protocols

    d. treatment protocols

2. Procurement of commodities

    NB vaccines & drugs should be on national formulary, from WHO approved manufacturer, and of proven quality

    a. vaccines

    b. drugs

    c. chemicals (e.g., lab reagents)

    d. diagnostics

    e. supplies (e.g., chlorine, soap, gloves, masks)

    f. equipment

3. Warehousing

    a. warehouse security

    b. complete storage of commodities in warehouse

    c. arrangements of pallets and shelves

    d. inventory system with stock cards—especially for drugs (SUMA)

    e. documentation of inflows and outflows

    f. central reporting

    4.   Distribution system (medical logistics)
       a.   product availability and price monitoring system
       b.   supervision of peripheral facilities
    5.   Provider training program for rational prescribing
    6.   Regulatory system
    7.   Issues summary

E. Health Information Systems

    1.   Vital
    2.   Clinical
    3.   Laboratory
    4.   Epidemiological
    5.   Financial
    6.   Issues summary

F. Health Financing

    1.   Subsidies
    2.   Costs, charges, and waivers
    3.   Provider incentives
    4.   Issues summary

G. Health Leadership and Governance

	MOH	PHO	DHO
1. Name			
2. Title			
3. Areas/programs of responsibility			
4. Working hours			
5. Communication methods			
6. Stated needs			
7. Organogram with contact list			
8. Issues summary			

References

1. UNICEF. Statistical tables. In: *The State of the World's Children*. New York: UNICEF, annual. Available from: http://www.unicef.org/sowc/.
2. WHO. Global Health Indicators. In: *World Health Statistics*. Geneva: World Health Organization, annual. Available from: the Global Health Observatory at http://www.who.int/gho/publications/world_health_statistics/en/.
3. US Centers for Disease Control and Prevention. (2001). Updated guidelines for evaluating public health surveillance systems—Recommendations from the Guidelines Working Group. *Morbidity and Mortality Weekly Report, 50*(RR–13), 1–35.

Tool 2.T2
EMERGENCY MANAGEMENT SYSTEM PROFILE

I.   EMERGENCY/DISASTER LEGISLATION AND POLICY

A.   **Statutory Definitions** (emergency, disaster, etc.)

B.   **Legal Assignment of Roles and Responsibilities for Disaster Management** (National Emergency Response Plan, National MCI Management Plan, Model State Emergency Health Powers Act)

1.   Disaster management authority
2.   Disaster warning and declaration
3.   Disaster plan activation
4.   Disaster command and control
5.   EOC/ICS stand-up and function
6.   Disaster assessment team(s) deployment
7.   Essential services provision
8.   Resource mobilization and management
   a.   technical assistance
   b.   material assistance (supply management)
   c.   financial assistance
   d.   volunteer assistance
   e.   coordination of assistance
9.   Authorities for drawing extra-budgetary funds in emergency operations
10. Authorities for appeal for external assistance (mutual aid agreements, etc.)
11. Public information
12. Contingency planning
13. Field reporting and restrictions

C.   **Special Emergency Powers** (protection of persons)

1.   Regulation of professionals (licensing, credentialing, privileging)
2.   Civil liability, immunity, and indemnification
3.   Protection from harms (workers' compensation)

D.   **Ad Hoc Advisories and Decrees**

1.   Law enforcement decrees (border control, curfew, lockdown, etc.)
2.   Health decrees (quarantine, burial, etc.)
3.   Immunization campaigns
4.   Personnel mobilization
5.   Customs procedures (drugs, supplies, equipment)

II.   COORDINATION OF AUTHORITIES

A.   **Lead Agency**

1.   Roles and responsibilities
2.   Locus of control
3.   Level and span of authority
4.   Full and part-time staff
5.   Chain of command
6.   Reporting methods
7.   Budget
8.   Other resources
9.   Policy
10. Programs

       11. Contingency plans
       12. Stated needs
       13. Reliability
       14. Organogram with contact list

  B.   **Stakeholders**

       1. Government
          a. central
          b. provincial/state
          c. local
       2. Ministries involved in disaster management
          a. civil defense
          b. foreign affairs
          c. communications
          d. transportation
          e. housing
          f. health
          g. hazard-specific agencies (seismology, etc.)
       3. Emergency services
          a. police
          b. fire
          c. ambulance
          d. hospitals
          e. others
       4. Military
       5. Private sector
          a. academia
          b. business
          c. community leaders
       6. UN agencies & IOs
       7. NGOs

  C.   **Mechanism of Coordination**

       1. Individual disaster preparedness activities
       2. Joint disaster preparedness activities
       3. MOU with other agencies or institutions
       4. Mutual aid agreements
       5. National program on disaster preparedness
       6. Field-based coordination

III. DISASTER PLANS—GENERIC ALL-HAZARDS

  A.   **Conceptual Framework**

       1. All hazards approach
          a. hazard-specific contingency plans
       2. Comprehensive approach (PPRR)
       3. Integrated (all agencies) approach
       4. Prepared community
       5. Resilient community

  B.   **Incident Management Principles**

       1. Common terminology
          a. organizational functions
          b. resource descriptions

      c.   incident facilities
2. Modular organization
3. Management by objectives
4. Incident action planning
5. Manageable span of control (3–7)
6. Incident facilities and locations
      a.   command posts
      b.   bases
      c.   staging areas
      d.   mass casualty triage areas
      e.   point of distribution sites
7. Comprehensive resource management
8. Integrated communications
9. Establishment and transfer of command
      a.   scope, jurisdiction, authority
      b.   standardized briefing at handover
10. Chain of command (orderly line of authority) and unity of command (all individuals have designated supervisor)
11. Unified command (allows agencies with different legal, geographic, and functional authorities to cooperate in multi-agency or multi-jurisdiction environment without compromising individual agency responsibility, authority, or accountability)
12. Accountability (of resources)
13. Dispatch/deployment (only on authorization and request)
14. Information management

C.   **Disaster Plan Development** (national/state/local/institutional)

1. Office(r) in charge of preparedness planning
2. Dedicated budget for preparedness planning
3. Planning scenarios

D.   **Disaster Plan Components**

1. Disaster authorities
2. Disaster warning and declaration
3. Disaster plan activation (levels)
4. Disaster command and control (ICS)
      a.   command (responsibility vs. authority)
      b.   operations
      c.   planning
      d.   logistics
      e.   finance
5. Emergency operations center
      a.   command (degree of autonomy)
      b.   SOPs
      c.   communications (interoperability)
      d.   site selection (accessibility)
      e.   support services (food, fuel, etc. for self-sufficiency)
6. Disaster assessment team(s) deployment
7. Essential services provision (scene operations)
      a.   command and control
      b.   communications
      c.   damage assessment
      d.   evacuation
      e.   firefighting
      f.   law enforcement, safety, and security
      g.   emergency health services provision

      h. shelter and mass care

      i. respite care

      j. secondary disaster prevention and hazard mitigation

      k. public information

          (1) information content

          (2) dissemination

          (3) media relations

          (4) special advisories and declarations

              (a)   health decrees (quarantine, burial, restrictions, bans, etc.)

              (b)   immunization campaigns

              (c)   personnel mobilization

              (d)   drug importation

  8. Recovery operations

  9. Resource mobilization (see VI)

      a. directory of key personnel

      b. inventory of critical resources

      c. spending authorities

IV.   DISASTER PLANS—HAZARD-SPECIFIC ANNEXES

A.   Natural Disasters

B.   Technological Disasters

C.   Conflict and Complex Emergencies

V.   DISASTER PLANS—HEALTH SECTOR-SPECIFIC FUNCTIONS (adapted from DHHS [1, 2])

A.   Preparedness of Community and Healthcare System

  1. Community

      a. determine risks to public health

      b. build community partnerships

      c. foster health-related social networks

      d. coordinate community engagement

  2. Healthcare system

      a. develop healthcare coalitions

      b. coordinate healthcare planning within the healthcare system

      c. prioritize essential healthcare assets and services

      d. identify gaps and mitigate them

      e. plan for at-risk groups with special needs

      f. coordinate training of healthcare workers

      g. conduct exercises and evaluation

B.   Emergency Operations Coordination

  1. Conduct preliminary assessment to determine need for disaster activation

  2. Activate public health emergency operations

      a. pre-identified key staff must respond in 60 min or less

  3. Develop incident response strategy

      a. incident action plan must be produced and approved before the start of the second operational period

  4. Manage and sustain the public health response

  5. Demobilize and evaluate public health emergency operations

C.   Public Health Surveillance/Epidemiological Investigation

  1. Conduct public health surveillance and detection

  2. Conduct public health and epidemiological investigations

3. Recommend, monitor, and analyze mitigation actions
4. Improve public health/epidemiological investigation systems

D. **Public Health Laboratory Testing**

1. Manage laboratory activities
2. Perform sample management
3. Conduct testing and analysis for routine and surge capacity
4. Support public health investigations
5. Report results

E. **Information Sharing**

1. Identify stakeholders to be incorporated into information flow
2. Identify and develop data elements and rules for sharing
3. Exchange information to determine a common operating picture

F. **Emergency Public Information and Warning**

1. Activate emergency public information system
2. Determine the need for a joint public information system
3. Establish and participate in information system operations
4. Establish avenues for pubic interaction and information exchange
5. Issue public information, alerts, warnings, and notifications

G. **Medical Surge**

1. Assess the nature and scope of the incident
2. Support activation of medical surge
3. Support jurisdictional medical surge operations
4. Support demobilization of medical surge operations

H. **Mass Care**

1. Determine mass care needs of the impacted population
2. Determine public health role in mass care operations
3. Coordinate public health, medical, and mental/behavioral health services
4. Monitor mass care population health

I. **Medical Countermeasure Dispensing**

1. Identify and initiate medical countermeasure dispensing strategies
2. Receive medical countermeasures
3. Activate dispensing modalities
4. Dispense medical countermeasures to identified population
5. Report adverse events

J. **Medical Materiel Management and Distribution**

1. Activate medical materiel management and distribution
2. Acquire medical materiel
3. Maintain updated inventory management and reporting
4. Establish and maintain security
5. Distribute medical materiel
6. Recover medical materiel and demobilize distribution operations

K. **Non-Pharmaceutical Interventions**

1. Engage partners and identify factors that impact non-pharmaceutical interventions
2. Determine non-pharmaceutical interventions
   a. personal hygiene
   b. isolation and quarantine

      c.   travel advisories and movement restrictions

      d.   social distancing

      e.   external decontamination

      f.   precautionary protective behaviors

   3. Implement non-pharmaceutical interventions

   4. Monitor non-pharmaceutical interventions

L. Responder Safety and Health

1. Identify responder safety and health risks
2. Identify safety and personal protective needs
3. Coordinate with partners to facilitate risk-specific safety and health training
4. Monitor responder safety and health actions

M. Volunteer Management

1. Notify volunteers needed and discourage those unneeded
2. Assemble, organize, and dispatch volunteers
3. Coordinate volunteers
4. Demobilize volunteers

N. Fatality Management

1. Determine role for public health in fatality management
2. Activate public health fatality management operations
3. Assist in the collection and dissemination of antemortem data
4. Participate in survivor mental/behavioral health services
5. Participate in fatality processing and storage operations

O. Community and Healthcare System Recovery

1. Community
   a. monitor health system recovery needs
   b. coordinate community health system recovery operations
   c. implement mitigation steps to limit future damages
2. Healthcare system
   a. develop healthcare system recovery processes
   b. assist implementation of continuity of operations planning

VI. DISASTER PLANS—MEDICAL LOGISTICS

A. Key Personnel Directory

1. Quantity, health discipline, and status (fit for duty, availability full-time, part-time)
2. Emergency mobilization
3. Deployment
   a. concentration point
   b. tasking orders
   c. materiel (clothing, PPE, supplies, equipment)
   d. transport
   e. telecommunications

B. Material Resources Inventory

1. Essential relief items (national list with specs and costs; local REA)
2. Sources
   a. existing supplies of essential relief items
   b. manufacturers/suppliers of essential relief items (local -> national)
   c. donations

3. Warehouses
   a. location
   b. size
   c. prepositioned resources (esp essential drugs, supplies, and EH items)
4. Tracking (SUMA)

C. **Transportation Systems** (land, sea, air)

1. Availability
2. Capacity
3. Costs
4. Key road entry/exit points
5. Fuel storage and distribution system

D. **Telecommunication Systems**

1. Country infrastructure
2. Government emergency communications center
   a. technologies
      (1) phone
      (2) fax
      (3) telex
      (4) e-mail
      (5) ham radio
      (6) satellite
   b. geographic range
   c. legal and technical restrictions on use
3. Disaster preparedness program communications center
4. Disaster management contact information
   a. national government
   b. MOH
   c. academic institutions, private sector
   d. donor organizations
   e. list of organizations operating in country (esp emergency response capacity)
   f. list of reference centers and resource persons with hazard-specific expertise
   g. community preparedness focal points

E. **Evacuation Planning**

1. Triggers
2. Routes
3. Shelters

F. **Program Budget**

1. Regular budget
2. Extra-budgetary (emergency operations)

References

1. US Centers for Disease Control and Prevention, Office of Public Health Preparedness and Response. (2011). *Public health preparedness capabilities: National standards for state and local planning*. Retrieved from www.cdc.gov/phpr/capabilities.
2. US Dept of Health and Human Services, Office of the Assistant Secretary for Preparedness and Response, and US Centers for Disease Control and Prevention, Office of Public Health Preparedness and Response. (2012). *Healthcare preparedness capabilities: National guidance for healthcare system preparedness*. Retrieved from http://www.phe.gov/preparedness/planning/hpp/pages/default.aspx.

Tool 2.T3
JURISDICTIONS

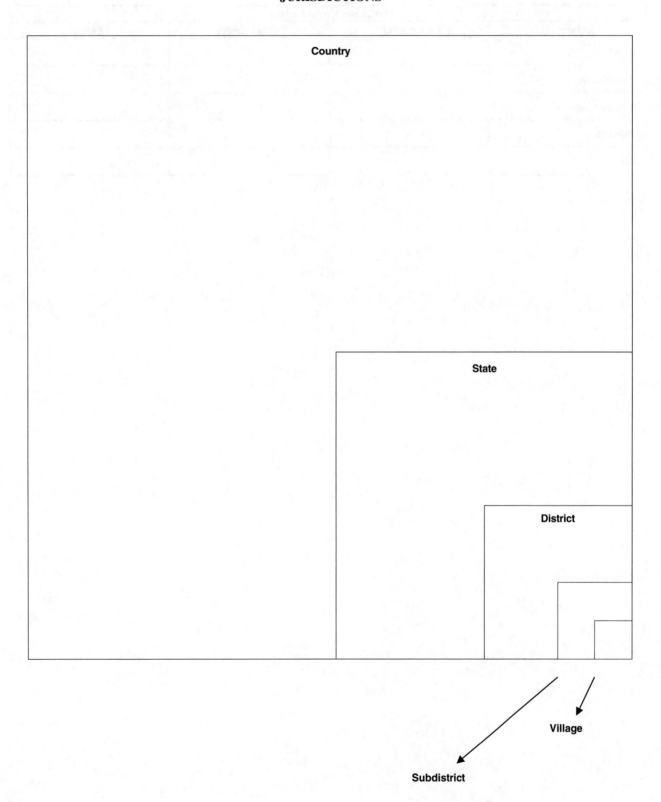

Health System Authorities

Health System Authorities			
Jurisdiction	**Government**	**Dept of Health**	**Clinical**
Central			
Province/State			
District/County			
Subdistrict			
Village			

Tool 2.T4
LAYERS OF CONFLICT

Faction	Leader	Geographic Stronghold	Size

Faction	vs. Faction	Issues

Tool 2.T4
CONFLICT CHRONOLOGY

Tool 2.T5
MEETINGS CALENDAR
Month: _____

	Mon		Tue		Wed		Thu		Fri		Sat		Sun
Date		**Date**		**Date**		**Date**		**Date**		**Date**		**Date**	
08:00													
10:00													
12:00													
14:00													
16:00													

Tool 2.T6
DISASTER RESPONSE CHRONOLOGY
Country, Year

	Disaster Events	Host Government, NDMA, Line Ministries	HCT & Partners	Donors (USAID, DFID, ECHO)
Jan				
Feb				
Mar				
Apr				
May				
Jun				
Jul				
Aug				
Sept				
Oct				
Nov				
Dec				

Contents

Glossary

ABX	antibiotics
ACAPS	Assessment Capacities Project
ACT	artemisinin-based combination therapy
AGR	annual growth rate
AR	attack rate
ARI	acute respiratory infection
BCC	behavioral change communication
BEOC	basic emergency obstetric care
CBR	crude birth rate
CBRNE	chemical, biological, radiological, nuclear, explosive
CD	communicable disease; complex disaster
CDC	Centers for Disease Control and Prevention (US)
CEOC	comprehensive emergency obstetric care
CERF	Central Emergency Response Fund (managed by OCHA)
CFR	case fatality rate
Cl	chlorine
CMR	crude mortality rate
CTC	community therapeutic care
d	day
DHF	dengue hemorrhagic fever
DHO	district health office

© David A. Bradt 2019
D. A. Bradt, C. M. Drummond, *Reference Manual for Humanitarian Health Professionals*,
https://doi.org/10.1007/978-3-319-69871-7_3

DM	diabetes mellitus
DPT	diphtheria, pertussis, and tetanus combination vaccine
DR	death rate
D_T	deaths total
E_0	life expectancy at birth
EHK	Emergency Health Kit
EOC	Emergency Operations Center
EPI	Expanded Programme on Immunization
FUO	fever of unknown origin
GAM	global acute malnutrition
GI	gastrointestinal
GIS	geographic information system
GNI	gross national income
GU	genitourinary
h	hour
HB	hepatitis B
HCW	health care worker
HDR	humanitarian daily ration
HeRAMS	Health Resources Availability and Mapping System
HF	hemorrhagic fever
HIS	health information system
HIV	human immunodeficiency virus
HPN	Humanitarian Practice Network
HTN	hypertension
IASC	Inter-Agency Standing Committee
ICS	incident command system
IDP	internally displaced person
IMCI	Integrated Management of Childhood Illness (WHO and UNICEF program)
IMPAC	Integrated Management of Pregnancy and Childbirth (WHO program)
IMR	infant mortality rate
IPC	Integrated Food Security Phase Classification
IPD	inpatient department
IPT	intermittent preventive treatment (of malaria)
IRA	initial rapid assessment
ITN	insecticide treated net
IYCF	infant and young child feeding
L	liter
L&D	labor and delivery
LBW	low birth weight
LDC	less developed country
m	meter
MIRA	multi-cluster initial rapid assessment
mL	milliliter
MMR	maternal mortality ratio
mo	month
MOH	Ministry of Health
MPS	Making Pregnancy Safer (WHO program)
MS	musculoskeletal
MSF	Médecins sans Frontières
MT	metric ton
NCD	non-communicable disease
NFI	non-food item
NGO	non-governmental organization

NTU	nephelometric turbidity units
O50	over 50 yrs of age
OCHA	Office for the Coordination of Humanitarian Affairs (UN)
OHCHR	Office of the High Commissioner for Human Rights (UN)
OPD	outpatient department
ORS	oral rehydration salts/solution
p	person
PDA	personal digital assistant
PDNA	post-disaster needs assessment
PEM	protein energy malnutrition
PHC	primary health care
PHO	provincial health office
PMTCT	prevention of mother-to-child transmission
PPE	personal protective equipment
P_T	population total
P_{T-pre}	population total pre-disaster
RH	reproductive health
RUTF	ready-to-use therapeutic food
SAM	severe acute malnutrition
SAR	search and rescue
SFP	supplementary feeding program
SGBV	sexual and gender-based violence
SPHC	selective primary health care
SRP	strategic response plan
SSA	Sub-Saharan Africa
STI	sexually transmitted infection
SUMA	supply management system (devised by WHO)
SWOT	strengths, weaknesses, opportunities, and threats
TFC	therapeutic feeding center
TFP	therapeutic feeding program
TFR	total fertility rate
TOR	terms of reference
U1	under 1 year-old
U5	under 5 year-old
U5MR	under 5 year-old mortality rate
U10	under 10 year-old
UNDAC	UN Disaster Assessment and Coordination
UNDP	UN Development Programme
UNHCR	UN High Commissioner for Refugees
UNICEF	UN Children's Emergency Fund
USAID	US Agency for International Development
VPI	vaccine preventable illness
WB	World Bank
WFP	World Food Programme (UN)
WHO	World Health Organization (UN)
wk	week
yr	year
Zn	zinc

Guidance Notes

Many assessments will occur in the post-disaster health sector. These include assessments of facility damage, medical logistics, health status, nutritional status, needs, hazards, probabilities, vulnerabilities, capabilities, risk, etc. Among the assessment instruments embraced by the IASC and the Global Health Cluster are Multi-Cluster Initial Rapid Assessment (MIRA), Health Resources Availability Mapping System (HeRAMS), as well as routine health information and disease surveillance systems. Current practice in international disaster relief calls for dedicated, non-operational actors (e.g. OCHA) to lead initial multi-party assessments and thereby inform operational decision-making of national governments and IASC Humanitarian Country Teams. This process is currently a mess. Numerous problems surround survey team leaders, issues in statistical representativeness, piloting of data gathering instruments, and complicated data management processes (e.g. use of PDAs to gather data, relational databases to aggregate the data, and SPSS to analyze the data). Overall, such assessments end up neither initial nor rapid, and ultimately of little use for early programmatic decision-making. In the acute disaster setting, this is doom.

Generic data collection forms should be standardized for the region and customized by parties to a (sub)national assessment. Such forms may already exist at MOH. If not, forms from external sources may be helpful though modifications may be needed and should be done in collaboration with the MOH. Forms should be simple with standard definitions and minimum essential data sets (MEDS) to avoid overburdening field workers. Field conditions are fluid, data are perishable, and informants are fickle. In collecting field data relevant for decision-making, several cardinal rules apply:

- Quick and dirty is better than slow and clean.
- The whole picture half right is better than half the picture wholly right.
- General accuracy is more important than statistical precision.
- Limited data are better than exhaustive data.
- Verified data are better than rumored data.
- Early is essential, and late is useless.

In the acute disaster setting, the only data that deserve collection are those that inform urgent field actions. Agencies may wish to collect additional data, but this should be done only if those data inform other critical decisions. Data gathering for academic researchers, report writing for agency donors, or media relations for advocacy groups are distractors early in a relief operation that divert attention from the operational focus of main effort.

There are three core Appendices in this section. They are intended for medical staff in a relief organization undertaking rapid epidemiological assessment (REA) in a specific catchment area in partnership with local providers. The REA (Document 3.1) is for overall assessment of the disaster-affected area. There are separate Appendices for assessment of specific sites (Document 3.2) and facilities (Document 3.3).

Rapid Epidemiological Assessment (Document 3.1)

Document 3.1 is one of the most versatile in the *Manual*. It is a data prompt and repository for pre-departure preparation, field briefing, field assessment, and field reporting. Consistent with the cardinal rules above, not all data are necessary at all times. However, the indicators listed have recurring relevance to the topic at hand. Selected comments about use of the Document in each of these phases of the mission follow below:

- **Pre-departure Preparation**

  Pre-existing indicators of the host country (Document 3.1, III elaborated in Tool 3.T1) can generally be uncovered pre-departure from listed sources. While the quantity of available indicators from these listed sources can be daunting, Tool 3.T1 focuses on key facts intelligible to field medical personnel, implementing agencies, and donor governments.

- **Field Briefing**

  Document 3.1 serves as a comprehensive, multi-sectoral repository for field data potentially provided by a broad array of sector specialists. Information chaos commonly prevails early in disaster, and a trusted data repository devised by the user can help master that chaos. Epidemiological data are particularly volatile with many different sources often competing with rumor. Tools 3.T2a, 3.T2b, and 3.T2c are very helpful in this context. So is a pencil.

- **Field Assessment**

  Document 3.1 presents tiered levels of detail in a modular structure. The tiered levels of detail facilitate expanded inquiry for areas of concern, or conversely allow limited inquiry for areas of little concern. The modular structure allows it to be broken apart for serial use by an individual or parallel use by partners. For example health sector function status (Document 3.1, VI) encompasses six major areas—public health services, clinical services, health workforce, medical logistics, health financing, and health leadership and governance. Staff may assess some or all of these areas with the appropriate component of the Appendix. Others sectors detail major determinants of health—security, water-sanitation, food, shelter, etc. Information from the assessment may not fully satisfy the professional dealing exclusively with a given subsector. However, the information is intended to satisfy the initial information needs of medical personnel and should enable informed discussion with the sector specialist.

- **Field Reporting**

  This is examined in detail in Section 5 of the manual.

Site-Specific Assessment (Document 3.2), **Feeding Center Assessment** (Document 3.3)

Documents 3.2 and 3.3 help to assess specific sites or facilities. The similarities in layout are self-evident. They are the results of a considered approach which uses:

- Serially preemptive information priorities—to enhance attention to critical issues
- Sector specific metadata—to enhance follow-up contact with key informants and reproducibility of findings
- Fixed data layout—to facilitate data entry
- SMART performance indicators with co-located benchmarks—to facilitate prompt interpretation of data collected
- Assessment form length limits of 2 pages—to enhance portability
- Time needed <2 h for one trained investigator in a population of 10,000 with knowledgeable, cooperative parties available for interview—to enhance utility

Findings from Documents 3.2 and 3.3 may be integrated into the broad scope of REA from Document 3.1. Serial use of Documents 3.2 or 3.3 in repeat visits to the field may help characterize developments at those sites. Additional exploration of the science behind REA may be found in the reference below [1].

Needs assessments should inform future action. They are often misused. They may be underutilized in mandate-driven decision-making of agencies and donors; they may be conducted by operational agencies to substantiate a request for funds; and they may be too slow to drive initial humanitarian response. Nonetheless, needs assessment remains a core skill of the medical coordinator. Conducting that assessment with lead agencies, host authorities, and operational partners is a corporate duty.

Reference

1. Bradt, D. A., & Drummond, C. M. (2002). Rapid epidemiological assessment of health status in displaced populations—An evolution toward standardized minimum essential data sets. *Prehospital and Disaster Medicine, 17*(4), 178–185. Corrected and republished in: (2003). *Prehospital and Disaster Medicine, 18*(1), 178–185.

Document 3.1
RAPID EPIDEMIOLOGICAL ASSESSMENT
Date

I. **INTRODUCTION** (copy A–B to Exec Summary)

    A. **Hazard History Abridged**

    B. **Current Disaster**

        1. When
        2. Who/what
        3. Where/extent
        4. Hazard magnitude/concentration/exposure time
        5. Mechanism of impact
        6. Secondary disaster (e.g. fire after earthquake, landslide after cyclone)
        7. Area affected
        8. Population affected

    C. **Immediate Response of Host Government Authorities**

        1. Disaster declaration
        2. Disaster plan activation
        3. Disaster command and control
        4. Emergency operations center
        5. Disaster assessment team(s)

    D. **Your Mission**

        1. Request by host authorities (person, position)
        2. Acceptance by your organization (person, position)
        3. Objectives (per TOR, examples below)
            a. assess disaster impact
            b. identify unmet needs in the health sector
            c. advise MOH/PHO/DHO of disaster impact and unmet needs
            d. recommend actions to prevent and/or control communicable diseases of epidemic potential
            e. assist with adaptation of normative technical best practices for local implementation
            f. plan goals, objectives, and projects for follow-up action by your agency
            g. provide on-site clinical care (substitution)
            h. provide on-site health sector coordination (substitution)
            i. monitor progress in disaster relief, rehabilitation, and recovery
            j. advocate with local and international donors for support of unmet needs of vulnerable populations
            k. contribute to local/regional health clusters or working groups as appropriate

II. **SOURCES AND METHODS**

    A. **Assessment Team Composition**

    B. **Assessment Area and Dates**

    C. **Information Sources and Assessment Methods**

        1. Review of secondary source data
            a. records and reports
            b. surveys and surveillance
            c. testimonies
            d. photographs and maps

2. Primary data gathered in structured and unstructured formats
   a. direct observation in site visits and transect walks
   b. key informant interviews
   c. convenience sampling of target population (e.g. community leaders, HCWs, members of vulnerable groups)
   d. focus (community) group discussions

D. **Logistics of Assessment Team**

E. **Constraints**

1. Security
2. Access
3. Transport
4. Telecommunications
5. Truth telling

III. **PRE-EXISTING INDICATORS** (summarize Tool 3.T1)

IV. **DISASTER IMPACT**

A. **Area Affected** (focus on most affected)

1. Geographic extent
2. Political jurisdictions (e.g. states, districts)

B. **Population Affected** (focus on most affected; see Tools 3.T2a and 3.T2b)

1. Population morbidity & mortality
   a. dead (rates generally not used for deaths from a single discrete event)
   b. injured
      (1) hospital admissions
         (a) evacuated
      (2) outpatients
   c. missing or unaccounted
2. Population undisplaced but crisis-affected
   a. accessible
   b. inaccessible/isolated
   c. host families (# or % of catchment population)
   d. total needing humanitarian assistance
3. Population displaced from usual homes   IDPs   refugees
   a. in organized camps or dispersed in camp-like settings
   b. in group accommodation apart from above
   c. in host families or individual accommodation
   d. new arrivals (specify time period)
   e. resettled
   f. total needing humanitarian assistance
4. Surviving vulnerable groups   IDPs   refugees
   a. U5
   b. malnourished
   c. orphaned
   d. abandoned
   e. pregnant
   f. lactating
   g. disabled
   h. elderly
   i. total needing humanitarian assistance

C. **Damage Assessment** (focus on most affected area; see Tool 3.T2c)

	destroyed	heavy damage	light damage
1. Material losses			

    a. homes

    b. commercial buildings

    c. industrial buildings

        (1) hazmat facilities

    d. public buildings

        (1) govt administration

        (2) hospitals

        (3) health centers

        (4) schools

        (5) community shelters

        (6) police stations

        (7) fire stations

	disrupted (%)	restored (%)
e. infrastructure/lifelines		

        (1) telecommunications

            (a) landlines

            (b) mobiles

            (c) satellite phones

            (d) radio net

            (e) internet

        (2) transportation network

            (a) roads

            (b) railroads

            (c) airports

            (d) seaports

        (3) utilities

            (a) electrical power supply

            (b) water supply

            (c) waste disposal

  2. Financial impact (PDNA)

    a. direct damages

    b. indirect losses

    c. impact on major sources of income (e.g. agriculture, industry)

D. **Secondary Disasters and Threats**

  1. Secondary phenomena (e.g. floods after storms)

  2. Hazard recurrence

  3. Weather complications and predictions

  4. Epidemics

  5. CBRNE consequences

  6. Areas of concern (e.g. flooding → gastroenteritis, hepatitis, leptospirosis, dengue, malaria, vipers)

E. **Disaster Impact Summary**

V. CURRENT EPIDEMIOLOGICAL INDICATORS

A. **Epidemiology**

  1. Mortality

    a. total deaths, excess mortality

    b. proportional mortality

        (1) cause-specific proportion of D_T (diarrhea, measles have each caused up to 40% of D_T in acute disasters)

        (2) D_T/P_T % (if $D_T \geq 1\%$ of P_T)

c.   death rates & trends
   (1)   crude (<1/10,000/d; >2 is critical)
   (2)   age-specific e.g. 0–5 DR (<2/10,000/d; >4 is critical) (often 50% of D_T)
   (3)   disease-specific (uncommonly used)
   (4)   excess (crisis death rate–baseline death rate)
d.   case-fatality ratios
   (1)   diarrhea (cholera 2–50%, dysentery 2–20%; target is CFR <1%)
   (2)   ARI (pneumonia 2–20%)
   (3)   malaria
   (4)   measles (2–30%)
   (5)   malnutrition (25–50% in SAM; associated with 50% of U5 deaths)
   (6)   trauma (20% of civilian injured in acute military conflict)

2.   Morbidity
   a.   total cases
   b.   proportional morbidity
      (1)   acute disease (epi estimates underlying early versions of EHK)
         (a)   adult presentations (1 adult obtains ~4 consults/yr; 5000 adults obtain ~5000 consults/3 mo)
                % adults presenting with: GI 25%, ARI 20%, MS 15%, GU 15%, malaria 10%, trauma 5%, anemia 5%, ocular 5%
         (b)   pedes (1 child obtains ~5 consults/yr; 5000 children obtain ~6500 consults/3 mo)
                % pedes presenting with: GI 30%, ARI 30%, worms 20%, malaria 15%, trauma 10%, anemia 10%, ocular 10%, otic 5%
      (2)   chronic disease (20% of P_T)
   c.   incidence rates & trends
      (1)   presentation rate/d (1% baseline–10% in CDs)
      (2)   age-specific (high risk = U5, O50)
      (3)   disease-specific (DART MMMM)
         (a)   **d**iarrhea (AR 50%/mo in U5 excluding below)
            (i)   dysentery (AR 5–30% over 1–3 mo in P_T)
            (ii)   cholera (AR 1–5% over 1–4 mo in P_T)
         (b)   **ARI** (AR 50%/mo in U5 esp in cold weather)
         (c)   **m**alaria (AR 50%/mo in P_T non-immune; 2%/mo in P_T immune (WHO))
                holo-endemic—intense transmission year-round (Congo)
                (6–10 infections/child/yr; mortality highest in U5 & preg F)
                hyper-endemic—intense transmission seasonally (W. Afr) (4–6 infections/child/yr; mortality across all ages)
                hypo-endemic—low transmission year-round (Thai-Burma)
                (1 infection/person/yr; mortality across all ages)
         (d)   **m**easles (AR 10%/epidemic in U12 non-immunized; 10–75% of cases with complications depending on health status)
         (e)   **m**alnutrition
            (i)   macro (PEM 10% with $Z < -2$, 1% with $Z < -3$)
            (ii)   micro (vitamins A–D; Fe, I)
         (f)   **t**rauma
            (i)   (para)military conflict
            (ii)   rape
            (iii) domestic violence
            (iv)   motor vehicle trauma
         (g)   **m**ental health
            (i)   adjustment disorders (debilitating grief reactions)
            (ii)   psychiatric disease (e.g. psychoses, affective disorders) (severe—baseline 2–3% of P_T + 1% increase post-disaster (net 50% increase); mild-mod—baseline 10% of P_T + 5–10% increase post-disaster (net 50–100% increase))
            (iii) violence
            (iv)   drug abuse

B. **Outbreaks and Epidemics**

   1. Recent or ongoing
      a. etiology
      b. date of first case(s)
      c. location
      d. number of cases or attack rate
      e. consequences or current status

   2. Potential (see REA IV D 6)
      a. wide geographic relevance
         (1) measles
         (2) cholera (dehydrating diarrhea)
         (3) shigella (bloody diarrhea)
         (4) meningococcus (meningitis)
         (5) hepatitis A, E (acute jaundice syndrome)
         (6) influenza
         (7) other
      b. specific geographic relevance
         (1) malaria
         (2) dengue
         (3) viral hemorrhagic fevers (e.g. yellow fever, lassa fever, dengue HF)
         (4) typhoid (FUO)
         (5) leishmaniasis
         (6) rare but significant (polio, typhus, plague)
         (7) vectors
         (8) vermin
         (9) vipers
      c. specific age groups
         (1) polio (acute flaccid paralysis)
         (2) neonatal tetanus

C. **Epidemiological Summary**

VI. **HEALTH SECTOR FUNCTIONAL STATUS**

A. **Public Health Services** (focus on service disruptions, adequacy)

   1. Disease prevention
      a. primary prevention
         (1) vaccine coverage rates for major antigens (EPI coverage rate >90%)
            (a) measles
            (b) DPT
         (2) vaccine stocks   quantity available   location
            (a) measles
            (b) DPT
            (c) polio
            (d) hepatitis B
            (e) other
         (3) cold chain adequacy
         (4) staff adequacy
         (5) transport adequacy
         (6) most recent campaign in area
            (a) location
            (b) dates
            (c) organizer
            (d) coverage
         (7) other VPIs of epidemic potential

      b.   communicable disease control programs   Y/N   issues
- (1) diarrhea
- (2) ARI
- (3) malaria
- (4) HIV
- (5) TB
- (6) other

2. Epidemiological surveillance system (CDC [1])
   - a. system objectives
     - (1) case detection (CDs, NCDs e.g. malnutrition)
     - (2) outbreak detection
     - (3) epidemic forecasting
     - (4) trend monitoring
     - (5) priority setting
     - (6) workload estimation
     - (7) resource targeting & health program activity
     - (8) intervention evaluation
   - b. health events/indicator conditions and case definitions
   - c. system components and flow chart of operations
     - (1) what is the population under surveillance?
     - (2) what is the time period of data collection?
     - (3) what data are collected (standardized forms)?
     - (4) who provides the data?
     - (5) how are data transmitted?
     - (6) how are data stored?
     - (7) who analyzes the data?
     - (8) how are data analyzed and how often?
     - (9) how often are reports generated?
     - (10) to whom are reports disseminated?
     - (11) how are reports disseminated?
   - d. level of usefulness (users of data and actions taken)
   - e. system attributes
     - (1) simplicity
     - (2) flexibility
     - (3) sensitivity
     - (4) reliability
     - (5) acceptability
     - (6) positive predictive value
     - (7) representativeness
     - (8) timeliness
   - f. system resource requirements (direct costs)
     - (1) personnel
     - (2) other (computer & office equipment, travel, training, mobile phone)

3. Epidemic preparedness and response
   - a. plan of action and coordinating committee
     - (1) public health incident command system (PHICS)
     - (2) cholera command and control center (C4)
   - b. clinical case definitions
   - c. case mgmt guidelines for communicable diseases with epidemic potential
   - d. outbreak mgmt protocol
     - (1) surveillance definitions
     - (2) alert thresholds
     - (3) rapid response teams to investigate case reports

        (4)   epidemic investigation kits to use

        (5)   specimens to collect

        (6)   labs to verify diagnosis (including sample sharing for confirmatory testing)

        (7)   patients to identify, isolate, and treat (inpatient and outpatient settings)

            (a)   isolation areas to organize

            (b)   treatments to plan

        (8)   contacts to trace and ? quarantine

        (9)   hotlines to use for notifiable diseases and rumor investigation

    e.   primary and secondary prevention

        (1)   infection control protocols

        (2)   commodities

            (a)   vaccines (e.g. measles, meningitis)

            (b)   drugs (e.g. prophylactic meds)

            (c)   chemicals (e.g. soap, Ca hypochlorite)

            (d)   supplies (e.g. chlorimetric and colimetric monitors)

            (e)   equipment (e.g. PPE)

    f.   resource prepositioning (stockpiles, supply chain)

    g.   information mgmt and crisis communication (media strategy)

        (1)   health authorities, WHO

        (2)   political authorities

        (3)   community leaders and public

            (a)   social mobilization

            (b)   hygiene promotion and health education

            (c)   behavioral change communication (BCC)

    h.   contingency planning for epidemic consequences

        (1)   provision of essential services (lifelines)

        (2)   corpse mgmt

4.   Health promotion

    a.   targeted diseases

        (1)   acute epidemic diseases

        (2)   chronic diseases—HTN, DM, HIV/TB, asthma

    b.   health promotion activities

        (1)   community health education

        (2)   provider education

5.   Health protection (if significant to disaster response)

    a.   air quality (e.g. wildfires, volcanic eruptions)

    b.   injury control

    c.   occupational health and safety

    d.   hazardous materials (e.g. chemical releases)

    e.   disaster risk reduction (e.g. safe hospitals)

6.   Issues summary

B.   **Health Facilities and Clinical Services** (focus on service disruptions, adequacy; see Tool 3.T2c)

	Mobile Clinics	Fixed Clinics	Health Centers	District Hospitals
1. Quantity				
2. Catchment population				
3. Access to facility				
4. Staffing				
a. quantity (~1/1000 p)				
b. skill mix				
5. Caseload (1–10% of catchment population/d)				
6. Bed capacity (10/10,000 p)				
7. Bed occupancy				

8. Referral load (10% of caseload)
9. Referral system
10. Clinical services
    a. departments/units (verify functioning of expected services)
        (1) clinical
             (a) OPD
             (b) IPD
             (c) L&D
             (d) surgery
             (e) other
        (2) dispensary
        (3) diagnostic lab
        (4) blood bank
        (5) radiology
    b. special services (verify quality of care)
        (1) child health
             (a) Expanded Programme on Immunization (EPI)
             (b) Integrated Management of Childhood Illness (IMCI)
             (c) child protection
        (2) reproductive health (20% of P_T are F 15–44 yr; 20% (4% of P_T) are pregnant, 20% (4% of P_T) are lactating)
             (a) identify RH lead agency
             (b) prevent and manage consequences of SGBV (15–20% lifetime incidence in SSA)
                  (i)   emergency contraception (post rape)
             (c) reduce HIV transmission
                  (i)   abstain, be faithful, use condoms (ABCs)
                  (ii)   standard precautions
                  (iii) treatment of STIs
                  (iv)   PMTCT
             (d) safe motherhood—basic & comprehensive emergency obstetric care
                  (i)   antenatal care
                  (ii)   professional midwifery
                  (iii) clean delivery
                  (iv)   essential newborn care
                  (v)   referral options
             (e) family planning
                  (i)   general contraception
        (3) trauma
             (a) (para)military conflict
             (b) rape
             (c) domestic violence
             (d) motor vehicle trauma
        (4) mental health
             (a) adjustment disorders (e.g. debilitating grief reactions)
             (b) psychiatric disease (e.g. psychoses, affective disorders) (severe—baseline 2–3% of P_T + 1% increase post-disaster (net 50% increase); mild-mod—baseline 10% of P_T + 5–10% increase post-disaster (net 50–100% increase))
             (c) violence
             (d) drug abuse

            (5)   chronic diseases (20% of P_T)
                  (a)   HTN
                  (b)   DM
                  (c)   HIV/TB
                  (d)   asthma
                  (e)   other

    c. standardized case management
            (1)   clinical case definitions
            (2)   treatment protocols (ORS+Zn, ABX, ACT, IPT, and ITN will save 75% of U5 deaths)
            (3)   other clinical protocols
                  (a)   standard precautions
                  (b)   injection safety
                  (c)   medical waste mgmt
            (4)   essential (standard) drugs and rational drug use
                  (a)   EHKs
                  (b)   specialty kits
            (5)   referral guidelines
            (6)   secondary prevention

    d. infection control
            (1)   dedicated staff
            (2)   hand washing facilities
            (3)   stocks of essential supplies (soap, gloves, masks, gowns)
            (4)   infection control protocols (medical waste mgmt, safe transfusion)
            (5)   compliance

11. Utilities
    a. power supply
    b. water supply
    c. excreta disposal/septic system

12. Issues summary

C.   **Human Resources** (focus on catchment area of interest)

	Available/10,000 p	Needed (quantity)

1. Basic (not vocationally trained)
    a. traditional birth attendant
    b. community health worker
    c. nurse's aide
    d. other applicable

2. Mid, High (vocationally trained)
    a. surgical/lab/pharmacy tech
    b. nurse
    c. midwife
    d. pharmacist
    e. doctor
    f. health facility administrator
    g. public health staff (identify)
    h. other applicable

3. Major areas with staff shortage
4. Reasons for staff shortage (e.g. security, migration, salary)
5. Issues summary

D. **Essential Medical Products and Technologies** (medical logistics)

    1. National standards
        a. essential medicines formulary
        b. standardized equipment per level of care
        c. diagnostic protocols
        d. treatment protocols
    2. Procurement of commodities
        NB vaccines & drugs should be on national formulary, from WHO approved manufacturer, and of proven quality
        a. vaccines
        b. drugs
        c. chemicals (e.g. lab reagents)
        d. diagnostics
        e. supplies (e.g. chlorine, soap, gloves, masks)
        f. equipment
    3. Warehousing
        a. warehouse security
        b. complete storage of commodities in warehouse
        c. arrangements of pallets and shelves
        d. inventory system with stock cards—especially for drugs (SUMA)
        e. documentation of inflows and outflows
        f. central reporting
    4. Distribution system
        a. product availability and price monitoring system
        b. supervision of peripheral facilities
    5. Provider training program for rational prescribing
    6. Regulatory system
    7. Issues summary

E. **Health Information System**

    1. Vital statistics
    2. Clinical
    3. Laboratory
    4. Epidemiological
    5. Financial
    6. Issues summary

F. **Health Financing** (disaster-specific)

    1. Subsidies
    2. Costs, charges, and waivers
    3. Provider incentives
    4. Issues summary

G. **Health Leadership and Governance**

		MOH	PHO	DHO
1.	Name			
2.	Title			
3.	Areas/programs of responsibility			
4.	Working hours			
5.	Communication methods			
6.	Stated needs			
7.	Organogram with contact list			
8.	Issues summary			

H. **Health Sector Functional Status Summary**

VII. OTHER SECTORS

A. Security

1. Disruption of public services
   a. telecommunications
   b. transportation
   c. fuel supplies
   d. public utilities
   e. refuse collection
   f. medical care
   g. education
2. Breakdown of law and order
   a. looting
   b. black markets
   c. riots and demonstrations
   d. road closures
   e. convoy procedures
3. Commercial shutdown
4. Discredited government
5. Military command and control
6. Frequent, widespread, or systematic armed violence
7. Incidents (impair access)

   NB access limited by weather, poor infrastructure, denial of permission to move, extortion, as well as overt security incidents

   a. crimes (International Criminal Court Rome Statute) (Article 5)
      (1) genocide (Article 6)

      acts committed with intent to destroy, in whole or in part, a national, ethnic, racial, or religious group

      (2) crimes against humanity (Article 7)

      acts committed as part of a widespread or systematic attack against any civilian population, with knowledge of the attack

      (3) war crimes (Article 8)
         (a) grave breaches of the Geneva Conventions of 12 Aug 1949
         (b) serious violations of laws and customs applicable in international armed conflict
         (c) serious violations of common article three applicable in non-international armed conflict (acts vs. persons taking no active part in the hostilities, including armed forces placed hors de combat by sickness, wounds, detention, or other cause)
         (d) non-applicability of (c) to internal disturbances (riots, sporadic violence, etc.)
         (e) other serious violations of laws and customs applicable in non-international armed conflict

      (4) crimes of aggression (provision to be adopted)

   b. other incidents
      (1) type
         (a) bombing and shelling
         (b) landmines
         (c) improvised explosive devices (IED)
         (d) unexploded ordnance (UXO)
         (e) sniping
         (f) chemical, biological, radiological (CBR) weapons
         (g) attacks on critical facilities
      (2) perpetrators
         (a) law enforcement (interior ministries, police)
         (b) host country military & paramilitary groups
         (c) rebel groups
         (d) armed extremists

     (e) armed gangs

     (f) street thugs

  8. Displacement (IDPs, refugees)

    a. reason

    b. reception/registration at new site

  9. Fears

    a. anniversary dates of violence

    b. fears of national staff

    c. fears in the community

    d. rumors of community violence

    e. rumors about activities of your agency

  10. Issues summary

B. **Protection** (who, where, from what)

  1. Security incidents (per REA VII A)

  2. Harmful traditional practices

    a. traditional tattoo centers

    b. female genital cutting

    c. gender-based violence

    d. early marriage

    e. forced marriage

    f. polygamy

    g. wife disinheritance

  3. Illegal commercial practices

    a. abduction

    b. trafficking (people, commodities, drugs)

    c. prostitution

    d. child labor with exposure to health and safety risks

  4. Non-commercial exploitative/abusive practices

    a. recruitment into armed forces

    b. sexual abuse

    c. child abuse

    d. spousal abuse

  5. Issues summary

C. **Safety** (for all parties to relief operation)

  1. Environmental hazards (e.g. natural hazards, falling debris)

  2. Street hazards (e.g. ground debris, vehicle traffic)

  3. Buildings (e.g. fire safety, structural integrity)

  4. Vehicles (e.g. seatbelts, road worthiness)

  5. Hazard mitigation activities

  6. Issues summary

D. **Search and Rescue** (if relevant to relief operation)

  1. Persons rescued

  2. Areas of activity

  3. Anticipated duration of SAR phase of relief operations

  4. Issues summary

E. **Logistics** (esp for relief agencies)

  1. Telecommunications

    a. landlines

    b. mobile phones

    c. satellite phones

    d. radio net

    e. internet

2. Transportation, fuel
   a. type
   b. availability
   c. cost
3. Issues summary

F. **Environment**

1. Climate and weather (exacerbations from seasonal weather, El Nino, climate change)
   a. temperature (heat load)
   b. precipitation
      (1) water storage status
      (2) drought-related restrictions
   c. wind, storms
2. Topography (altitude, terrain, natural hazards)
3. Edaphic factors (soil type, surface water presence, rain water drainage, flora, fauna e.g. vermin, snakes, infestations)
4. Impacts
   a. site-specific impacts (if focal, give details; if widespread, highlight major aspects)
      (1) present owner
      (2) original use
      (3) overall area (45 m²/p)
      (4) road access
      (5) water access & drainage (1–6% slope—rise over run)
      (6) site hazards (e.g. ordnance, toxic waste)
      (7) hazard mitigation feasibility
   b. agriculture impacts
      (1) cropping cycle
      (2) planting status, seed supplies, water supplies
      (3) harvest status
      (4) market availability of produce
      (5) current prices
   c. livestock impacts
      (1) animal nutrition status
      (2) stock rearing
      (3) stock selling
      (4) market availability of animals
      (5) current prices
   d. livelihood impacts
      (1) farmers
      (2) pastoralists
      (3) manufacturers
   e. clinical impacts (particularly where relevant to program service delivery and beneficiary morbidity)
      (1) vectors
      (2) diseases
5. Issues summary

G. **Environmental Health**

1. Water
   a. sources available & outputs (in order of preference)
      (1) aquifers (deep preferred to shallow)
         (a) wells
         (b) handpumps
         (c) boreholes
      (2) surface water (flowing preferred to still)
         (a) still
         (b) flowing

      (3)   fixed storage tanks & bladders

      (4)   trucks

      (5)   other

  b.   access (250 p/water point, <500 m from housing)

  c.   distribution/collection method

  d.   queue time (<15′)

  e.   quantity (5 L/p/d initially → 15–20 L/p/d after 60 d)

  f.   quality

      (1)   sources of contamination

         (a)   open storage containers

         (b)   excreta (latrines, septic tanks)

         (c)   dumpsites

         (d)   chemical storage facilities (e.g. fuel depots)

      (2)   purification method (at source & end user levels)

      (3)   water testing method & results

         (a)   0 coliforms/dL

         (b)   0.05 mg/dL free Cl

         (c)   <5 NTU (nephelometric turbidity units) (if hand is visible immersed in water, NTU < 5)

2.   Sanitation

    NB describe site cleanliness, types of waste, magnitude of problem, collection methods & frequency, disposal methods & site, special issues (e.g. waste separation) for:

  a.   excreta (50–100 p/latrine initially → 20 p/latrine after 60 d, 30 m from housing, 100 m from H_2O)

  b.   household waste

      (1)   garbage

      (2)   sullage

  c.   solid waste

  d.   medical waste

      (1)   sharps

      (2)   biologics (e.g. placentas)

      (3)   paper/plastic, dressings, bandages

  e.   corpses

  f.   dead animals

3.   Food

    NB describe overall food security in integrated phase classification (IPC) terms with attention to following major dimensions

  a.   availability/adequacy

      (1)   quantity (2100 kcal/p/d min with 10–12% from protein, 17% from fat, plus micronutrients from fresh or fortified foods)

      (2)   variety

      (3)   market proximity to settlements

  b.   access (purchasing ability)

  c.   utilization

      (1)   food hygiene

      (2)   cooking

         (a)   equipment availability

         (b)   fuel type & availability

         (c)   preparation—family vs. communal

  d.   market stability and resilience

      (1)   inflation

      (2)   exchange rates

      (3)   market performance

         (a)   price seasonality

         (b)   price volatility

    e.   altered livelihood and coping strategies
- (1) livestock sales
- (2) firewood & charcoal sales
- (3) self-employment
- (4) labor migration
- (5) decreased consumption of preferred foods (skipping meals)
- (6) increased consumption of wild foods
- (7) gifts & remittances
- (8) school truancy
- (9) commercial sex work
- (10) organized crime

    f.   distributions and targeted feedings (IPC 3+, if U5 GAM >10%)
- (1) blanket supplementary feeding program (SFP)
- (2) targeted supplementary feeding program
- (3) community therapeutic care (CTC)
- (4) therapeutic feeding program (TFP)

4. Shelter and settlements
    a.   shelter
- (1) building materials, construction techniques (e.g. prefab), and quality
- (2) covered space ($3.5 \text{ m}^2/\text{p}$; 2 m between shelters)
- (3) adequacy of weather protection
- (4) evidence of damages

    b.   settlements (build environment)
- (1) locations
- (2) security and safety
- (3) hazard risks (e.g. fire in camps)
- (4) emergency/contingency planning for risks
- (5) access to communication links, transportation hubs
- (6) community density (p/km^2)
- (7) community leaders identified

5. Emergency relief supplies (non food items)
    a.   plastic sheeting
    b.   blankets
    c.   jerry cans
    d.   cooking utensils
    e.   hygiene kits
    f.   mats
    g.   ITN

6. Vector/vermin/vipers, reservoirs
    NB describe type of vectors, magnitude of presence, disease risks, control methods, special issues (e.g. breeding sites, reservoir management)
    a.   mosquitoes
    b.   rodents
    c.   other

7. Public utilities
    a.   power supply
    b.   water supply
    c.   waste disposal/septic system

8. Issues summary

VIII.   RESPONSE OF DOMESTIC (HOST COUNTRY) AUTHORITIES

  A.   **Disaster Management Mechanism**

     1.   Disaster management authority
     2.   Disaster warning and declaration
     3.   Disaster plan activation
     4.   Disaster command and control
     5.   EOC/ICS stand-up and function
     6.   Disaster assessment team(s) deployment
     7.   Essential services provision
     8.   Resource mobilization and management
        a.   technical assistance
        b.   material assistance (supply management)
        c.   financial assistance
        d.   volunteer assistance
        e.   coordination of assistance
     9.   Domestic donations
     10. International appeals (stated needs of health authorities)
     11. Public information (press releases, websites)
     12. Contingency planning
     13. Field reporting and restrictions

  B.   **Emergency Protection Powers in Disasters** (model legislation)

     1.   Regulation of professionals—licensing, credentialing, privileging
     2.   Immunity, indemnification, and civil liability of providers
     3.   Protection of workers from harm—exposure limits, compensation

  C.   **Advisories and Decrees**

     1.   Law enforcement decrees (emergency, border control, curfew, etc.)
     2.   Health decrees (quarantine, burial, etc.)
     3.   Immunization campaigns
     4.   Personnel mobilization
     5.   Customs procedures (drugs, supplies, equipment)

  D.   **Issues Summary**

IX.   RESPONSE OF INTERNATIONAL COMMUNITY

  A.   **Coordination of International Assistance**

     1.   HCT
     2.   UNDAC
     3.   HC
     4.   Cluster system
        a.   health cluster

  B.   **Intervenors**

     1.   Stakeholder analysis (brief SWOT analysis)
        a.   GOs
        b.   UN
        c.   IOs
        d.   NGOs
     2.   Geographic areas of activity
     3.   Domains of activity

C. **Multi-party Assessments**

    1. Types
        a. (M)IRA
        b. HeRAMS
        c. HIS
    2. Gaps—unmet needs (see Tools 3.T3a and 3.T3b)

D. **International Appeals** (OCHA Financial Tracking Service)

    1. Flash
    2. CERF
    3. SRP

E. **Issues Summary**

    1. [Needs − (Coping Strategy + Assistance) = Unmet Needs]

X. **RESPONSE OF REPORTING AGENCY** (delete if assessment is multi-party or single purpose undertaking without operational follow-up)

A. **Assessment Activities Undertaken**

B. **Assistance Projects/Activities Undertaken** (range of options below)

    1. Reallocation of existing local & national resources
    2. Revision/refinement of present (medical) practices
        a. use of essential drugs
        b. use of standardized case management
        c. elimination of dated practices
    3. Financial assistance (critical funding)
    4. Technical assistance (critical skills)
        a. complement donated goods
        b. support appropriate technology
        c. develop information systems
    5. Material assistance (critical goods)
        a. essential drugs and vaccines
        b. consumable supplies
        c. other stated needs of health authorities
    6. Direct service provision (substitution)
    7. Coordination of external assistance
    8. Capacity building of host authorities
    9. Civil society partnership and support
        a. organize community leaders
        b. encourage gender mainstreaming
        c. encourage privatization
        d. discourage entitlements
    10. Advocacy
    11. Transition to early recovery
    12. Monitoring and evaluation

XI. **OPERATIONAL CONSTRAINTS**

A. **Security**

B. **Political/Administrative**

C. **Logistical**

D.   **Technical**

E.   **Economic**

F.   **Developmental**

XII.   **REA PRINCIPAL FINDINGS AND ANALYSIS** (copy to Exec Sum; list major findings from section summaries; emphasize summaries bolded below as most relevant to health sector; delete headings if simpler to serially list findings; use phrases, not sentences)

A.   **Disaster Impact Summary** (see REA IV E)

B.   **Epidemiological Summary** (see REA V C)

C.   **Health Sector Functional Status Summary** (see REA VI H)

D.   Security, Protection, and Safety (see REA VII A, B, C)

E.   Search and Rescue (see REA VII D)

F.   Logistics (see REA VII E)

G.   Environment (see REA VII F)

H.   **Environmental Health** (see REA VII G)

I.   **Stated Needs of Health Authorities** (see REA VIII A10)

J.   **Major Gaps** (see REA IX E)

K.   **Operational Constraints** (see REA XI)

L.   Duration of Emergency Phase (see REA VIII C1)

M.   Future Risk Factors and Scenario Forecasting (see REA IV D)

Reference

1. US Centers for Disease Control and Prevention. (2001). Updated guidelines for evaluating public health surveillance systems—Recommendations from the Guidelines Working Group. *Morbidity and Mortality Weekly Report, 50*(RR-13), 1–35.

Document 3.2
SITE-SPECIFIC ASSESSMENT

Date _____   Assessor _____

Site Name _____   Informant #1 _____

Location—GPS/landmark _____   Informant #2 _____

Population   registration Y N   total pop_____   # households   _____

U1 _____ (5%)   women (15–44) _____ (20%)   arrivals/wk   _____

U5 _____ (20%)   men (15–44) _____ (10%)   departures/wk   _____

5–14 _____ (35%)   45+ _____ (15%)   typical livelihood _____

vulnerable groups _____

Security   Officer in Charge _____   Camp Leader _____

Indicators   incidents at site Y N type (murder, rape, assault) _____

Issues   _____

Site Mgmt   Lead Agency _____   Contact _____   Ph/Fax _____

Indicators   original site use _____   area (m²) _____   area (m²/p) _____ (>45)

road access   OK   not OK   problem _____

water availability   OK   not OK   problem _____

drainage   OK   not OK   problem _____

building repair   OK   not OK   problem _____

electricity   OK   not OK   problem _____

Issues   _____

Water   Lead Agency _____   Contact _____   Ph/Fax _____

Indicators   site sources _____   open hours/d _____

\# wells _____   # bladders/tanks _____   # taps or h. pumps _____

condition of units _____   user fees Y N amount _____   p/tap or h. pump _____ (<250, 500)

m to home _____ (<500)   # users waiting _____   queue time (′) _____ (<30)

home sources _____   10–20 L sm neck containers Y N overall L/p/d _____ (>15)

turbid Y N   color Y N   odor Y N

chlorination Y N   how _____   fecal coli/100 mL _____ (0)

Issues   _____

Sanitation Lead Agency _____   Contact _____   Ph/Fax _____

Indicators   \# latrines _____   # full or blocked _____ (0)   p/usable latrine _____ (<20)

latrine type and grouping _____   squat plate Y N

visible feces Y N   m from ground H_2O _____ (>30)   m from dwelling _____ (<50)

handwash points Y N   type (tap, bucket)   soap gm/p/mo _____ (>250)

cleaning supplies Y N   maintenance teams Y N   printed health messages Y N

wash bucket Y N   p/communal basin _____ (<100)   showers Y N

refuse drums Y N   families/drum _____ (<10)   waste pit—dwelling (m) _____ (<100)

vermin/vectors Y N   type _____   eradication activities Y N

Issues   _____

Food/Nutrition Lead Agency _____   Contact _____   Ph/Fax _____

Indicators current foods _____   kcals/p/d _____ (>2100)

household stores Y N   recent changes Y N   food security Y N

food income (5 sources)   crops Y N   livestock Y N

labor exchange Y N   wild foods Y N   relief Y N

cash income (5 sources)   crops Y N   livestock Y N

labor Y N   borrowing Y N   selling other assets Y N

food distribution Y N   type, quantity, frequency _____

markets with food Y N   communal kitchen Y N   family kitchen & fuel Y N

Issues   _____

Non-Food Lead Agency _____   Contact _____   Ph/Fax _____

Indicators mats/mattresses Y N   blankets Y N   kitchen sets Y N

hygiene parcels Y N   warehoused supplies Y N   kinds _____

Issues   _____

Shelter Lead Agency _____   Contact _____   Ph/Fax _____

Indicators # tents _____   # buildings _____   building materials _____

sheeting Y N   bednets used Y N   shelter m^2/p _____ (>3.5)

Issues   _____

Health Lead Agency _____   Contact _____   Ph/Fax _____

Indicators clinic on site Y N   time/distance from camp _____   days/hours open _____

structure ok Y N   # doctors _____ # nurses _____   # CHWs _____   # TBAs _____

running water Y N   toilet/latrine Y N   electricity Y N

exam rooms _____   ORS corner Y N   overnight stay Y N

dispensary Y N   drug shortages Y N   IV fluid Y N

sharps container Y N   med waste disposal _____   handwashing Y N

comms Y N   referral transport Y N   treatment fees Y N

standard case defs Y N   treatment protocols Y N   stats reporting Y N

case definition simple diarrhea _____

treatment simple pedes diarrhea _____   ORS prep demonstrated Y N

patients understand mechanism of diarrhea transmission Y N

total visits/wk _____   active case finding Y N   % total pop/d _____ (<1)

total deaths/wk _____   active death finding Y N   deaths/10k p/d _____ (<1)

total referrals/wk _____   referral destination _____   diseases referred _____

Total # cases simple diarrhea _____   dysentery _____   visually confirmed Y N

(past wk) ARI _____   how diagnosed _____   (respiratory rate)

measles _____   cold chain present Y N   date of last campaign _____

malaria _____   how diagnosed _____   falciparum Y N

malnutrition _____   type _____   nutrition program Y N

trauma _____   type _____

psych _____   fear in population Y N   reason _____

disease outbreaks Y N   type & date _____   epidemic control plan Y N

provider stated needs _____

Issues   _____

Community Priorities   **Assessor Priorities**

1. _____   1. _____

2. _____   2. _____

3. _____   3. _____

Document 3.3
FEEDING CENTER ASSESSMENT

Date _____   Assessor _____

Site Name _____   Informant #1 _____

Location—GPS/landmark _____   Informant #2 _____

Population   registration Y N   total pop _____   # households   _____

U1 _____ (5%)   women (15–44) _____ (20%)   arrivals/wk   _____

U5 _____ (20%)   men (15–44) _____ (10%)   departures/wk   _____

5–14 _____ (35%)   45+ _____ (15%)   typical livelihood _____

vulnerable groups _____

Security   Officer in Charge _____   Camp Leader _____

Indicators   incidents at site Y N type (murder, rape, assault) _____

Issues   _____

Site Mgmt   Lead Agency _____   Contact _____   Ph/Fax _____

Indicators   original site use _____   area (m²) _____   area (m²/p) _____ (>45)

road access   OK   not OK   problem _____

water availability OK   not OK   problem _____

drainage   OK   not OK   problem _____

building repair   OK   not OK   problem _____

electricity   OK   not OK   problem _____

Issues   _____

Water   Lead Agency _____   Contact _____   Ph/Fax _____

Indicators   site sources _____   open hours/d   _____

\# wells _____   # bladders/tanks _____   # taps or h. pumps _____

condition of units _____   user fees Y N amount _____   p/tap or h. pump   _____ (<250, 500)

m to home _____ (<500)   # users waiting _____   queue time (′)   _____ (<30)

home sources _____   10–20 L sm neck containers Y N   overall L/p/d   _____ (>30)

turbid Y N   color Y N   odor Y N

chlorination Y N   how _____   fecal coli/100 mL _____ (0)

Issues   _____

Sanitation   Lead Agency _____   Contact _____   Ph/Fax _____

Indicators   # latrines _____   # full or blocked _____ (0)   p/usable latrine   _____ (<20)

latrine type and grouping _____   squat plate Y N

visible feces Y N   m from ground H₂O _____ (>30)   m from dwelling   _____ (<50)

handwash points Y N   type (tap, bucket)   soap gm/p/mo   _____ (>250)

cleaning supplies Y N   maintenance teams Y N   printed health messages Y N

wash bucket Y N   p/communal basin _____ (<100)   showers Y N

refuse drums Y N   families/drum _____ (<10)   waste pit—dwelling (m) _____ (<100)

vermin/vectors Y N   type _____   eradication activities Y N

Issues   _____

Nutrition Lead Agency _____ Contact _____ Ph/Fax _____

Indicators

date opened _____ hours open _____ staffing _____

admission criteria _____

current phase 1 census	U5 _____	O5 _____	Total _____
current transition census	U5 _____	O5 _____	Total _____
current phase 2 census	U5 _____	O5 _____	Total _____
admissions last wk	U5 _____	O5 _____	Total _____
cumulative admissions	U5 _____	O5 _____	Total _____

trend analysis _____

coverage _____ (rural > 50%, urban > 70%, camp > 90%) active case finding Y N

estimated unmet needs _____

medical protocol Y N reference_____

    hypoglycemia, hypothermia — D10 or F75

    ABC (dehydration, sepsis) — ReSoMal or RL + D5 or ORS

    GI (feeds) — F75 (initial), F100 +/− solid food (recovery)

    ID (3) — antibiotics (TMP/SMZ), antihelminths (mebendazole), +/− antimalarials

    adjuncts — vitamins A-D, minerals, measles vaccine, Fe (only in rehab phase)

underlying illnesses malaria Y N % _____ TB/HIV Y N % _____

referrals out Y N number last wk _____ destination _____

discharge criteria _____

disposition _____

cure rate _____ (>75%) death rate _____ (<10%) default rate _____ (<15%)

provider stated needs _____

Issues _____

Health Lead Agency _____ Contact _____ Ph/Fax _____

Indicators

clinic on site Y N	time/distance from camp _____	days/hours open _____
structure ok Y N	# doctors _____ # nurses _____	# CHWs _____ # TBAs _____
running water Y N	toilet/latrine Y N	electricity Y N
exam rooms _____	ORS corner Y N	overnight stay Y N
dispensary Y N _____	drug shortages Y N	IV fluid Y N
sharps container Y N	med waste disposal _____	handwashing Y N
comms Y N	referral transport Y N	treatment fees Y N
standard case defs Y N	treatment protocols Y N	stats reporting Y N

case definition simple diarrhea _____

treatment simple pedes diarrhea _____ ORS prep demonstrated Y N

patients understand mechanism of diarrhea transmission Y N

total visits/wk _____ active case finding Y N % total pop/d _____ (<1)

total deaths/wk _____ active death finding Y N deaths/10k p/d _____ (<1)

total referrals/wk _____ referral destination _____ diseases referred _____

Total # cases (past wk)

simple diarrhea _____	dysentery _____	visually confirmed Y N (respiratory rate)
ARI _____	how diagnosed _____	
measles _____	cold chain present Y N	date of last campaign _____
malaria _____	how diagnosed _____	falciparum Y N
malnutrition _____	type _____	nutrition program Y N
trauma _____	type _____	
psych _____	fear in population Y N	reason _____
disease outbreaks Y N	type & date _____	epidemic control plan Y N

provider stated needs _____

Issues _____

Community Priorities

1. _____

2. _____

3. _____

Assessor Priorities

1. _____

2. _____

3. _____

Tool 3.T1
PRE-EXISTING INDICATORS

A. **Population Affected**

1. Census (may be simplified as <5 yr and ≥ 5 yr)

	M	F	Total

    a. <1
    b) 1–4
    c) 5–14
    d) 15–44
    e) ≥45
    f) total

2. Demography
    a. race, ethnicity, religion
    b. languages
    c. socioeconomic status
    d. urban vs. rural
    e. average family/household size

B. **Settlements**

1. Overall size of affected area
2. Locations
    a. community size, geographic separation
    b. access to transportation hubs and communication links
3. Population mobility
4. Community density
    a. geographic separation of families within the settlement
5. Shelter type and quality
6. Hazard exposure (e.g. upcoming seasonal natural hazards)
7. Equality/discrimination within the community
8. Conflict within the community
9. Emergency preparedness
10. Known coping mechanisms

C. **Access to Essential Services** (see UNICEF [1], WHO [2] for country data)

1. Public utilities (infrastructure)
    a. % with improved water
    b. % with improved sanitation
    c. % with electricity
    d. % with telephones/television
2. Health services
    a. skilled health care workers (all)/10,000 p   (23)
    b. physicians/10,000 p   0.2)
    c. nurses/10,000 p   (1)
    d. midwives/10,000 p   (1)
    e. community health workers/10,000 p   (10)
    f. % population with provider coverage   (100%)
    g. consultations/p/yr   (1)
    h. % pregnancies receiving antenatal care   (100%)
    i. % deliveries attended by trained staff   (90%)
    j. % immunization rates—measles vac in 1 yr/o   (90%)
    k. hospital beds/10,000 p   (10)
    l. health facilities with BEOC, CEOC/500,000 p (4, 1)
    m. admissions/10,000 p
3. Underserved areas (by location and type of service)

D.   **Health Status** (see UNICEF [1], WHO [2] for country data)

   1.   Mortality and other rates
      a.   CBR   (10–50)
      b.   CMR   (5–25)
      c.   AGR   (%)
      d.   IMR   (3–200)
      e.   U5MR   (3–300)
      f.   MMR   (5–2100)
      g. E_0 at birth M/F/T (40–85)
      h.   TFR   (2–8)

   2.   Nutritional status
      a.   caloric intake/p/d (2100 kcal)
      b.   % infants with low birth weight (LBW) (7% with <2.5 kg)
      c.   % U5 with growth faltering (30%)
      d.   % U5 with global acute malnutrition (GAM) (10%)
      e.   % with micronutrient deficiencies (vitamins A-D; Fe, I)
      f.   % of food supply from international food assistance (WFP, NGOs)

   3.   Endemic diseases
      a.   HIV prevalence
      b.   TB prevalence
      c.   malaria incidence
      d.   other major diseases

   4.   Health beliefs and traditions
   5.   Sources of care
   6.   Referral system

E.   **Macroeconomic Status** (see UNICEF [1], UNDP [3], WB [4] for country data)

   1.   Labor force occupations
      a.   agriculture
      b.   pastoralism
      c.   industry
      d.   services

   2.   Unemployment rate
   3.   GNI per capita ($US)
   4.   Inflation rate
   5.   % population in extreme poverty (<$1.90/d income)
   6.   Gini index (Gini coefficient × 100 expressed as %) (0–100)
   7.   Public spending as % of GDP allocated to health (1–10)
   8.   Central government expenditures on health as % of total govt expenditure
   9.   Per capita government expenditure on health at average exchange rate
   10. Per capita total expenditure on health at average exchange rate

F.   **Educational Status** (see UNICEF [1] for country data)

   1.   Adult literacy rate
   2.   Female literacy rate

G.   **Developmental Status** (see UNDP [3] for county data)

   1.   Human development index
   2.   Fragile states typology (USAID)
      a.   post-conflict transition
      b.   early recovery
      c.   arrested development
      d.   deterioration

References

1. UNICEF. Statistical tables. In: *The state of the world's children*. New York: UNICEF, annual. Available from http://www.unicef.org/sowc/.
2. WHO. Global health indicators. In: *World health statistics*. Geneva: World Health Organization, annual. Available from the Global Health Observatory at http://www.who.int/gho/publications/world_health_statistics/en/.
3. United Nations Development Programme. Statistical annex. In: *Human development reports*. New York: UNDP, annual. Available from http://www.hdr.undp.org/en.
4. World Bank. *World development indicators*. Washington, DC: World Bank, annual. Available from http://wdi.worldbank.org/tables.

Tool 3.T2a

ESTIMATES OF DISASTER-AFFECTED POPULATION

Source: Ministry of _____, Capital City

Date _____

Location	Population per census of ___ year	Population Undisplaced		Population Displaced			Missing or unaccounted	Injured	Dead
		Accessible	Inaccessible or isolated	IDPs	Refugees	Total			
Needing HA (# or %)									
Total									

Tool 3.T2b

ESTIMATES OF DISASTER-AFFECTED VULNERABLE GROUPS

Source: Ministry of _____, Capital City

Date _____

Vulnerable groups in location	Total number	Population Undisplaced		Population Displaced			Missing or unaccounted	Injured	Dead
		Accessible	Inaccessible or isolated	IDPs	Refugees	Total			
U5									
Malnourished									
Orphaned									
Abandoned									
Pregnant									
Lactating									
Disabled									
Elderly									
Needing HA (# or %)									
Total									

Tool 3.T2c
DAMAGE ESTIMATES

Source: Ministry of _____, Capital City

Location _____   Date _____

Structure	Preexisting	Damaged			Functional (# or %)
		Destroyed	Heavy	Mod-Light	
Residential					
Commercial					
Industrial					
Hazardous Materials					
Subtotal or %					
Public Bldgs					Functional (# or %)
Govt Admin					
Hospitals					
Health Centers					
Schools					
Community Shelters					
Police Stations					
Fire Stations					
Subtotal or %					
Lifelines					% Population with access
Telecomms Landlines Mobiles					
Transport Road Rail Air					
Power supply					
Water supply					
Septic system					

Tool 3.T3a
SECTORAL GAP IDENTIFICATION

Function	Site 1	Site 2	Site 3	Site 4
Site Management				
Protection/Registration				
Security				
Logistics and Transport				
Water				
Sanitation				
Food Aid				
Non-Food Aid				
Shelter				
Health				
Education and Training				
Early Recovery				
Other				

Tool 3.T3b

HEALTH SECTOR GAP IDENTIFICATION

Function	Site 1	Site 2	Site 3	Site 4
Sector Management				
Immunization				
Clinical Health Services Health Center/Post				
Clinical Health Services Mobile clinics				
Clinical Health Services Hospital				
Clinical Pathology Laboratory support				
Special Services Reproductive health				
Special Services Maternal-child health				
Special Services Mental health				

Special Services HIV/AIDS				
Special Services Nutrition				
Epidemic Preparedness				
Communicable Disease Control				
Community Health Education				
Epidemiological Surveillance				
Medical Logistics				
Other				
Other				

Field Recommendations

4

Contents

Guidance Notes

Disasters are complicated environments. Recommendations fall prey to many feasibility traps—technical, administrative, political, economic, and developmental among them. Moreover, temporary solutions tend to become permanent. While there seems not enough time to do things properly at the outset, there is apparently enough time to do them over and over again. Hence, disaster decision-making requires impulse control and considered thought before action. Fortunately, most relief interventions are well-established. There are few silver bullets. Different organizations, e.g., Medecins Sans Frontieres, and Humanitarian Policy Network, have published lists of generic priority interventions. For the disaster medical coordinator, several points are emphasized below.

- Health determinants extend well beyond the health sector per se. Security and environmental health are critical loci of health determinants. An attempt to define disaster health priorities, even for a single organization, must recognize the importance of these extra-sectoral origins of health determinants.
- "Unmet needs" is a core concept that devolves from quantifying needs offset by coping strategy and ongoing assistance. You cannot manage what you cannot measure, and if you cannot measure, you cannot quantify.
- Information is an essential disaster relief commodity—an anxiolytic which must be managed as diligently as therapeutic goods.
- Public health interventions generally save the most lives and are the most cost-effective. They are the first health sector priority in disasters.
- Clinical interventions in disasters may have little evidence for cost-effectiveness. Among them are certain platforms for donor response—foreign disaster medical assistance teams, foreign field hospitals, and hospital ships—which usually arrive too late to contribute significantly to the relief effort. Even in natural disasters yielding high numbers of trauma patients, such as earthquakes, the international experience (typified by Gujarat, Bam, Jogyakarta, Port-au-Prince, etc.) shows the burden of acute trauma care redistributes quickly, local providers do most of the work, and imported facilities become underutilized. Indeed, the facilities imported to provide acute trauma care often become millstones of the relief community—expensive, resource intensive, and poorly integrated with the local health system. Among successful field surgical teams, the ICRC generalist approach to war surgery is most compelling—basic surgical tools, basic surgical

© David A. Bradt 2019
D. A. Bradt, C. M. Drummond, *Reference Manual for Humanitarian Health Professionals*,
https://doi.org/10.1007/978-3-319-69871-7_4

principles, no specialist surgeons, no onward referral. When dealing with individual patients, it's most helpful to ask one more question and do one fewer test.

- Beware of malpractice in disaster relief operations:
  - programmatic decisions without multi-party needs assessment
  - programmatic interventions without beneficiary input
  - non-reporting/non-sharing of local epidemiological data
  - non-participation in health sector/cluster coordination processes
  - health services without environmental health
  - clinical care without proper medical waste disposal
  - noncompliance with standardized case management
  - early primary closure for contaminated traumatic wounds
  - antidepressants for PTSD diagnosed in the field
  - introduction of unsustainable technology
  - establishment of refugee camps
  - population abandonment (under cover of "program transfer" to local health authorities) once international media leave and funding ends
  - glowing reports of program success which rely on process indicators without impact/outcome indicators

Rapid Epidemiological Assessment Recommendations (Document 4.1)

Document 4.1 contains a set of draft recommendations applicable to a broad range of settings in an "all hazards" environment. The recommendations are consistent with the conceptual framework, yet remain sensitive to disaster health determinants outside the health sector. The recommendations encompass the field as well as "upstream" issues that may require action at headquarters level. Although these recommendations appear context-free, sectional summaries from the REA in the field will inform the choice of specific actions.

Recommendations should appear in priority order, ideally number fewer than a dozen, and be concisely reported on one page. The Recommendations Summary Worksheet (Tool 4.T1) may help organize the medical coordinator's thinking. Beneficiary unmet needs, agency mandate, political pressures, and resource availability may all influence the exact priority of recommendations submitted. Nonetheless, multi-party needs assessments should drive field responses, and recommendations should reflect beneficiary unmet needs. State them candidly and clearly. Above the medical coordinator in the organization's chain of command, no one else will have more insight or legitimacy in characterizing those needs.

Document 4.1
RAPID EPIDEMIOLOGICAL ASSESSMENT RECOMMENDATIONS
Date

XIII. RECOMMENDATIONS (copy to Exec Summary)

A. **Information Priorities**

    1. Security information (protection issues)
    2. Safety information (hazard issues)
    3. Intervenor information (4 Ws)
    4. REA information (health sector issues)
    5. GIS data (location issues)
    6. WASH subsector analysis
        a. water (tanker) distribution system
        b. water quality testing findings
        c. HH water storage findings
    7. Food security subsector analysis
        a. VAM (WFP), IPC, or FEWS NET analysis
        b. pipeline analysis
        c. market analysis
        d. transfer modality analysis
    8. Health subsector surveys & surveillance
        a. epidemiological surveillance (EWARS, q 1 wk)
        b. health facilities and provider survey (HeRAMS, q 3 mo)
        c. nutritional survey (U5 WHZ, q 6 mo)
        d. immunization survey (U5 EPI, annual)
        e. communicable disease control survey (disease-specific)
        f. vector survey (presence, speciation, pathogen detection, eradication plan)
        g. medical logistics survey

B. **Health Intervention Priorities** (activities, not objectives)

Top 10 generic priorities recommended by other sources:

List 1   initial assessment, measles immunization, water and sanitation, food and nutrition, shelter and site planning, health care, control of communicable diseases and epidemics, public health surveillance, human resources and training, coordination (MSF [1])

List 2   adequate shelter, sufficient safe food, sufficient safe water, sanitation facilities, environmental sanitation and waste disposal, mass vaccination, primary health care and referral care, disease surveillance and outbreak control, vector control, and health education and social mobilization (HPN [2])

    1. Public health services
        a. disease prevention
            (1) primary prevention
                (a) measles immunization (6 mo–12 yr (MSF); 6 mo–5 yr (CDC); coverage > 90%)
                    (i) vaccine stocks
                    (ii) cold chain
                (b) vitamin A distribution
                (c) restart EPI
            (2) communicable disease control (CDs of epidemic potential)
                (a) diarrhea
                (b) ARI
                (c) malaria

(d) HIV

(e) TB

(f) other

b. epidemiological surveillance (key data on health status, nutritional status, or health program activity)

  (1) data sources

    (a) provider-based alert system (24 h notice for notifiable conditions)

    (b) camp-based weekly system (esp from larger camps > 2500 p)

    (c) facility-based weekly system (from IPDs and OPDs)

    (d) lab-based weekly system (isolation and identification)

    (e) other relevant epi data—rumor and outbreaks

  (2) surveillance system components

    (a) clinical case definitions

    (b) camp logbooks

    (c) weekly surveillance report forms

    (d) reporting process—description and diagram

c. epidemic preparedness and response

  (1) plan of action and coordinating committee

    (a) public health incident command system (PHICS)

    (b) cholera command and control center (C4)

  (2) clinical case definitions

  (3) case mgmt guidelines for communicable diseases with epidemic potential

  (4) outbreak mgmt protocol

    (a) surveillance definitions

    (b) alert thresholds

    (c) rapid response teams to investigate case reports

    (d) epidemic investigation kits to use

    (e) specimens to collect

    (f) labs to verify diagnosis (including sample sharing for confirmatory testing)

    (g) patients to identify, isolate, and treat (inpatient and outpatient settings)

      (i) isolation areas to organize

      (ii) treatments to plan

    (h) contacts to trace and ? quarantine

    (i) hotlines to use for notifiable diseases and rumor investigation

  (5) primary and secondary prevention

    (a) infection control protocols

    (b) commodities

      (i) vaccines (e.g., measles, meningitis)

      (ii) drugs (e.g., prophylactic meds)

      (iii) chemicals (e.g., soap, calcium hypochlorite)

      (iv) supplies (e.g., chlorimetric and colimetric monitors)

      (v) equipment (e.g., PPE)

  (6) resource prepositioning (stockpiles, supply chain)

  (7) information mgmt and crisis communication (media strategy)

    (a) health authorities, WHO

    (b) political authorities

    (c) community leaders and public

      (i) social mobilization

      (ii) hygiene promotion and health education

      (iii) behavioral change communication (BCC)

            (8)   contingency planning for epidemic consequences
                (a)   provision of essential services (lifelines)
                (b)   corpse mgmt

    d.   health promotion (relevant to disaster response)
        (1)   targeted diseases
            (a)   acute epidemic diseases
            (b)   chronic diseases—HTN, DM, HIV/TB, asthma
        (2)   health promotion activities
            (a)   community health education
            (b)   provider education

    e.   health protection (relevant to disaster response)
        (1)   air quality (e.g., wildfires, volcanic eruptions)
        (2)   injury control
        (3)   occupational health and safety
        (4)   hazardous materials (e.g., chemical releases)
        (5)   disaster risk reduction (e.g., safe hospitals)

2.   Health facilities and clinical services

    a.   vulnerable groups (IDPs on the move > IDPs in camps > IDPs in host communities > host country nationals staying put)

    b.   access to care

    c.   clinical epidemiology
        (1)   ID
            (a)   diarrhea
            (b)   ARI
            (c)   malaria
            (d)   measles
            (e)   epidemic diseases
        (2)   malnutrition
        (3)   trauma
        (4)   mental illness
        (5)   chronic diseases

    d.   delivery of health services
        (1)   stabilize and evacuate critical patients
        (2)   restore workforce (staff need to care for their own families)
            (a)   redistribute host country staff
            (b)   use task shifting
            (c)   encourage incentives (recognition, benefits, payments)
            (d)   provide health situation updates for providers
        (3)   initiate/restore levels of care and referral system
            (a)   home visiting by CHWs referring to health clinic
                (i)   active case finding
                (ii) ORS and soap distribution
                (iii) referral for immunization and key clinical symptoms
                (iv) health education
                (v) defaulter follow-up
            (b)   mobile clinics referring to fixed clinic
            (c)   fixed clinics referring to health center
            (d)   health centers referring to district hospital
            (e)   emergency medical teams & foreign field hospitals linked to referral system

(4)   initiate/restore primary, preventive, and basic services
    (a)   comprehensive primary health care (focusing on community-based interventions, health education, and standardize case management)
        (i)   SPHC as needed in severe resource-limited settings
    (b)   child health services
        (i)   EPI
        (ii)   IMCI
        (iii)   protection
    (c)   reproductive health services
        (i)   identify RH lead agency
        (ii)   prevent and manage consequences of SGBV (IASC Guidelines)
            (a)   emergency contraception (post rape)
        (iii)   reduce HIV transmission (IASC Guidelines)
            (a)   abstain, be faithful, use condoms (ABCs)
            (b)   standard precautions
            (c)   treatment of STIs
            (d)   PMTCT
        (iv)   safe motherhood—basic & comprehensive emergency obstetric care (IMPAC programs)
            (a)   antenatal care
            (b)   professional midwifery (midwifery kits)
            (c)   clean delivery (clean delivery kits)
            (d)   essential newborn care (warming and exclusive breast feeding)
            (e)   referral options
        (v)   family planning—plan for comprehensive RH services in PHC
            (a)   general contraception
    (d)   trauma services
        (i)   field stabilization
        (ii)   evacuation
        (iii)   initial facility care including damage control surgery
        (iv)   inter-hospital referral & definitive care
        (v)   rehabilitation
        (vi)   cost recovery
    (e)   mental health services (IASC Guidelines & Action Sheets)
        (i)   coordination
        (ii)   assessment, monitoring, & evaluation
        (iii)   protection & human rights standards
        (iv)   human resources
        (v)   community support
        (vi)   health services
        (vii)   education
        (viii)   dissemination
    (f)   chronic diseases (prioritize resource requirements beyond EHKs)
(5)   reinforce standardized case management
    (a)   clinical case definitions
    (b)   treatment protocols (ORS+Zn, ABX, ACT, IPT, and ITN will save 75% of U5 deaths)
    (c)   other clinical protocols
        (i)   standard precautions
        (ii)   injection safety
        (iii)   medical waste mgmt
    (d)   essential (standard) drugs and rational drug use
        (i)   EHKs, National Pharmaceutical Stockpile push packs
        (ii)   specialty kits (including chronic disease kit)

         (e)   referral guidelines

         (f)   secondary prevention

     (6)   reinforce infection control

         (a)   dedicated staff

         (b)   hand washing facilities

         (c)   stocks of essential supplies (soap, gloves, masks, gowns)

         (d)   infection control protocols (medical waste mgmt, safe transfusion)

3. Human resources
   a. areas and services in need
   b. sources of staff
   c. salaries/incentives for staff
   d. security for staff
4. Essential medical products and technologies (medical logstics)
   a. national formulary
   b. warehouse security
   c. storage of commodities completely in warehouse
   d. arrangements of pallets and shelves
   e. inventory system with stock cards—especially for drugs (SUMA)
   f. documentation of inflows and outflows
   g. central reporting
   h. supervision of peripheral facilities
   i. monitoring of aid distributions
5. Health information systems
   a. vital statistics
   b. clinical
   c. laboratory
   d. epidemiological
   e. financial
6. Health financing
   a. subsidies
   b. costs, charges, and waivers
   c. provider incentives
7. Health leadership and governance
   a. key leaders
   b. technical support to coordination process

C. Other Sectoral Intervention Priorities

1. Security
   a. strategy
      (1) locate refugees/IDPs > 20 km from borders and conflict areas
      (2) declare humanitarian corridors, pauses, and cease-fires
      (3) separate military from civilians (cantonment), and militias from non-combatants
      (4) disarm combatants (especially near refugees/IDPs)
      (5) demobilize military, disband militias (especially near refugees/IDPs)
      (6) repatriate, reintegrate former combatants in society of origin
      (7) arrest and prosecute perpetrators of violence
   b. military/police operations as needed
      (1) duty posts
      (2) checkpoints
      (3) patrols
      (4) escorts
      (5) safe havens

(6)   search and seizure of weapons

(7)   non-combatant evacuation

(8)   civil-military cooperation

    (a)   central coordination

    (b)   agreement on responsibilities and objectives

    (c)   common territories of responsibility

    (d)   compatible communications

    (e)   collocation

    (f)   liaison

    (g)   inter-agency meetings

    (h)   routine contacts between desk officers

    (i)   civil-military operations centers

    (j)   joint reconnaissance and assessments

2.   Protection (who, where, from what)

  a.   actors

    (1)   civilian lead protection agency (UNHCR, OHCHR, OCHA)

      (a)   monitor protection violations

      (b)   document protection violations—incident lists, spot maps, and trend analysis

      (c)   report events of concern to local authorities

      (d)   review with host government

      (e)   ensure follow-up

    (2)   intervenor credentialing

    (3)   refugees/IDPs

      (a)   self-organization

      (b)   go and see visits (respected refugee/IDP leaders visit country/area of origin)

      (c)   come and talk visits (respected leaders from country/area of origin visit refugees/IDPs)

  b.   protective programming

    (1)   maintain access to refugees/IDPs (protection by presence)

    (2)   register refugees/IDPs

    (3)   reunify families and undertake child tracing

    (4)   establish community watch (no relocations without consent)

    (5)   ensure refugees/IDPs participate in program decisions

    (6)   deploy dedicated protection officers

    (7)   identify the most vulnerable

    (8)   advocate for the most vulnerable

      (a)   confirm

      (b)   document

      (c)   mobilize (share info with third parties who can influence authorities)

      (d)   persuade (directly with authorities)

      (e)   publicize

      (f)   stigmatize

      (g)   denounce

    (9)   establish spaces and services for the most vulnerable without stigmatization

      (a)   child-friendly spaces

      (b)   women's centers

      (c)   psychosocial services

   (10) beware of economic implications

      (a)   reimbursement schemes for injury & death (which disfavor the illiterate and remote)

      (b)   reimbursement schemes for land damages (which favor large landowners over tenant farmers and squatters)

      (c)   land tenure issues for widows

      c. health diplomacy (Health as a Bridge for Peace)

- (a) humanitarian pauses
- (b) humanitarian corridors
- (c) medevac
- (d) safe spaces, conflict exclusion zones
  - (i) immunization days
  - (ii) food distributions
  - (iii) NFI distributions
  - (iv) verification visits

3. Safety (for all parties to relief operation)
   a. personal protective equipment (PPE)
   b. hazard-specific mitigation plans (see also C6)
4. Search and rescue (if ongoing)
5. Logistics (esp for relief agencies)
   a. telecommunications plan
   b. transportation, fuel
6. Environment
   a. site-specific mitigation plans (see also C3)
   b. site stabilization, drainage (with understanding of local conditions during seasonal weather changes)
7. Environmental health
   a. water supply
      (1) sources—near the people if possible; if not, bring it to the people rather than people to it. Aquifer > surface water.
         (a) if aquifer—deep > shallow
         (b) if surface—flowing > still
      (2) access—monitor it vs. patrol it vs. guard it
      (3) quantity (5 L/p/d initially → 15–20 L/p/d after 60 d)
         (a) bucket distribution with hand chlorination
         (b) jerry cans (20 L) with hand chlorination
         (c) tanker trucks (8000 L) with chlorinated water
         (d) water bladders (3000–10,000 L) with chlorinated water (500 p/d served by 10 MT bladder; 10 k p need 200 k L/d from 10 × 10 MT bladders filled 2×/d)
         (e) wells → handpumps (serve 500 p/d, require bucket chlorination) → submersible pumps (serve 5 k p/d, enable batch chlorination)
         (f) boreholes with pumps > surface water treatment units
         (g) piped systems
      (4) quality (0 coliforms/dL)
         (a) source protection (esp wells)
            (i) separate surface water and defecation areas
            (ii) fence to keep out animals
            (iii) wall to keep out children
            (iv) cover to keep out adults
            (v) container which doesn't touch ground
            (vi) channel to run-off spills
         (b) storage system protection
            (i) cover on jars and jerry cans
            (ii) personal hygiene
         (c) water purification (0.05 mg/dL free Cl, < 5 NTU)
            (i) physical (boiling, filters—ceramic, sand, compressed clay + rice husk)
            (ii) chemical (chlorination, alum flocculation; tankers vs. on-site storage cisterns vs. hand chlorination of household jerry cans and buckets)
            (iii) radiological UV (SODIS)

          (iv) combination (portable water purification units with filtration, flocculation, and chlorination—15,000 L/h)

          (v) reverse osmosis

b. sanitation

  NB priority populations: new & existing IDP camps > IDPs in urban areas & host communities where existing facilities are over taxed > rural communities with IDP returns

  (1) excreta disposal

    (a) facilities construction (50–100 p/latrine initially → 20 p/latrine after 60 d, <50 m from housing, >30 m from H_2O)

      (i) defecation fields (days)

      (ii) trench latrines (weeks)

      (iii) public pit latrines (weeks) (1 M p need 20 k latrines on 20 k m^2 space)

      (iv) family pit/raised latrines (depends on water table) (months)

      (v) pour flush (siphon) toilets (months)

      (vi) septic system (year)

    (b) hand hygiene

      (i) water points and soap (250 g bathing soap/p/mo, 200 g laundry soap/p/mo)

    (c) hygiene promotion

    (d) operations and maintenance

      (i) maintenance teams

      (ii) cleaning supplies

  (2) garbage disposal

    (a) collection and removal

    (b) burial

  (3) solid waste disposal

    (a) incineration

    (b) burial

  (4) medical waste disposal

    (a) incineration

    (b) burial

  (5) corpse management

    (a) disaster victim identification

    (b) disposal

      (i) cremation

      (ii) burial

  (6) dead animal management

    (a) incineration

    (b) burial

c. food and nutrition

  (1) beneficiary population (IPC 3+, GAM > 5%)

  (2) assistance target (% of above)

  (3) assistance ration (% of MDR; 50% is common for WFP)

  (4) transfer modality

    (a) food (general food distribution)

    (b) food for assets (formerly food for work)

    (c) cash

    (d) voucher

  (5) general food distribution

    (a) commodity basket standardization (based on family size and HIV status)

    (b) mechanism (0.5 kg/p/d, 15 kg/p/mo, 1 MT/1000 p/2 d, 15 MT/1000 p/mo, 450 MT/10,000 p/3 mo, 30,000 MT (prepo depot size)/2 M p/mo)

  NB plan depends on population distribution, disaster damage, security situation, and food distribution sites

(i)   humanitarian daily ration airdrops (Phase 1)

(ii) bulk foods by helicopter (Phase 2)

(iii) bulk foods by road (Phase 3)

(6) infant and young child feeding (IYCF)

(7) emergency school feeding (ESF)

(8) supplementary feeding program (>350 kcal/p/d with RUSF—Plumpy'Sup®, high energy biscuits; priorities are U5 (6 mo–5 yr) with GAM, pregnant (esp third trimester) or lactating women (esp first yr), medical referrals) (Sphere)

(a) blanket SFP if GAM > 20% or > 10% if aggravating factors

(b) targeted SFP if GAM > 10% or > 5% if aggravating factors

coverage goals: > 50% in rural areas, > 70% in urban areas, > 90% in camp settings (Sphere)

cure rate > 75%, CFR < 3%, defaulter rate < 15% (Sphere)

aggravating factors = CMR > 1/10,000/day, basic ration inadequate, epidemic communicable disease, or severe cold

NB   no SFP if GAM < 5%

(9) therapeutic feeding program (where SAM > 2%, GAM > 10%; GAM > 15% is critical) (WHO)

(a) TFC census should be < 50 (WHO); if > 50, add another site

cure rate > 75%, CFR < 10%, defaulter rate < 15% (Sphere)

(10) market interventions to ensure food affordability

(11) inspection (regulatory control over farms, abattoirs, and restaurants)

d. shelter & settlements (emergency shelter → transitional shelter → permanent housing)

(1) household shelter (in chronological order)

(a) 1–3 mo: emergency shelter in place (salvaged materials, plastic sheeting, tarpaulins > tents (think outside the tent))

(b) 3–12 mo: hazard-resistant transitional shelter (rehabilitated shelter > prefabricated shelter b/c $300 to buy, $300 to ship)

(c) 12 mo +: permanent housing built back better (cement floor with corrugated sheet metal sides & roofing)

(2) settlement options

(a) safe (home) site, same structures repaired

(b) safe (home) plot, emergency or transitional shelter

(c) host family

(d) resettlement in safe proximity to destroyed home

(e) resettlement in planned site (community/civic centers, schools, churches) for those without options a–d

(f) resettlement in camps (always last choice)

(3) shelter package (if relief/rehab distribution is needed)

(a) shelter repair kit, vouchers, or cash

(b) non-food items

(c) food basket

(d) assisted utilities

(e) debris removal

(f) tents (always last choice)

(4) settlement development (if reconstruction solution can be staged)

(a) wat/san

(b) transportation hubs, communication links

(c) homes, shop-homes

(i)   1 family = 5 people

(ii) 16 families = 80 people = 1 community

(iii) 16 communities = 1250 people = 1 block/village

(iv) 4 blocks = 5000 people = 1 sector

(v)   4 sectors = 20,000 people = 1 camp

        (d)   shops, stalls, and kiosks
        (e)   health facilities
        (f)   other civil buildings
    (5)   plan for permanent shelter using DRR best practices
        (a)   hazard-resistant design
        (b)   training in hazard-resistant construction
        (c)   public information campaigns on building back better

  e. emergency relief supplies (non food items)
    (1)   plastic sheeting
    (2)   blankets
    (3)   jerry cans
    (4)   cooking utensils
    (5)   hygiene kits
    (6)   mats

  f. vector control/reservoir control
    (1)   mosquitoes
        (a)   insecticide treated nets
        (b)   indoor residual spraying at beginning of transmission season (more effective in Asia than Africa; not appropriate for dengue)
        (c)   drainage/elimination of breeding sites
        (d)   larvicide in standing water
    NB   aerial spraying, outdoor spraying (fogging) are not really useful
    (2)   rodents
        (a)   food storage
        (b)   garbage disposal

8. Additional common concerns
  a. public utility restoration
    (1)   power supply
    (2)   water supply
    (3)   excreta disposal/septic systems

  b. resource prepositioning
    (1)   resource type
    (2)   feasibility of sourcing it
    (3)   feasibility of transporting, storing, and protecting it

  c. relocation (if security, environment, or environmental health incompatible with local human habitation)
    (1)   impact study (esp on land use and socio-economic issues in receiving areas)
    (2)   formal plan with contingency plan to scale back in event of problems
    (3)   government led coordination body to establish minimum standards
    (4)   donors and implementing partners involved in planning and agreed on standards
    (5)   informed consent
    (6)   family unification
    (7)   reciprocal visits prior to relocation (reps to sending and receiving areas) with information campaign to avert rumor
    (8)   basic infrastructure in place prior to relocation (feeder roads, water points, health clinics, schools)
    (9)   safe transport to resettlement sites with transit centers en route
    (10) safety net for settlers
        (a)   cash or food rations until next harvest (donor will not want this)
        (b)   land enabling agricultural self-sufficiency
        (c)   draft animals, seeds, and tools on grant basis
        (d)   social services for settlers and local communities
    (11) external monitoring

D.   **Coordination Priorities**

1.   Cluster/sector dedicated full-time coordinator
2.   NGO co-lead
3.   Cluster SAGs and TWiGs
4.   Inter-cluster working group
5.   Engagement and participation
     a.   HCT
     b.   local authorities
     c.   local NGOs
     d.   donors
     e.   beneficiaries (always retain capacities in terms of relationships, skills, values, norms, and decision-making processes)
6.   Cluster work products
7.   Humanitarian programme cycle deliverables and operational tempo
8.   L3 scale up
9.   Rapid response teams to assess and deliver
10. Contingency planning
11. Peer review
     a.   Operational Peer Review (OPR) (90 d) and L3 transitions
     b.   Emergency Directors' Group site visits
     c.   Inter-agency Humanitarian Evaluation (12 m)

E.   **Program Implementation**

1.   Reallocation of existing local & national resources
2.   Revision/refinement of present (medical) practices
     a.   use of essential drugs
     b.   use of standardized case management
     c.   elimination of dated practices
3.   Financial assistance (critical funding)
4.   Technical assistance (critical skills)
     a.   complement donated goods
     b.   support appropriate technology
     c.   develop information systems
5.   Material assistance (critical goods)
     a.   essential drugs and vaccines
     b.   consumable supplies
     c.   other stated needs of health authorities
6.   Direct service provision (substitution)
7.   Coordination of external assistance
     NB cooperation = shared goals; coordination = shared tasks; collaboration = shared resources
     a.   identification and registration of actors
     b.   actor/area/activity (who/what/where) matrix
     c.   gap analysis and priority setting
     d.   establishment of rapid response mechanism
     e.   gap filling via complementary inputs linking iNGOs & local NGOs to local health authorities
          (1)   technical—staff mobilization
          (2)   material—resource prepositioning and supply chain linkages
          (3)   financial—external resource mobilization
     f.   identification of deliverables and timetables
     g.   consolidated reporting and dissemination
          (1)   group terms of reference
          (2)   meeting minutes

       (3) epidemiology updates
       (4) health sitreps
       (5) component analysis
       (6) field documentation (toolkit) for new arrivals
8. Capacity building of host authorities
9. Civil society partnership and support
   a. organization of community leaders
   b. encourage gender mainstreaming
   c. encourage privatization
   d. discourage entitlements
10. Advocacy
11. Transition to early recovery

References

1. Médecins Sans Frontières. (1997). *Refugee health—An approach to emergency situations.* Hong Kong: Macmillan Education.
2. Checchi, F., Gayer, M., Grais, R. F., & Mills, E. J. (2007). Public health in crisis-affected populations—A practical guide for decision-makers. *Humanitarian Practice Network, Network Paper No 61, December 2007.* London: Overseas Development Institute.

Tool 4.T1
RECOMMENDATIONS WORKSHEET

A. **Information Priorities**

B. **Health Intervention Priorities**

  1. Public health services
  2. Health facilities and clinical services
  3. Human resources
  4. Essential medical products and technologies
  5. Health information systems
  6. Health financing
  7. Health leadership and governance

C. **Other Sectoral Intervention Priorities**

  1. Security
  2. Protection
  3. Safety
  4. Search and rescue
  5. Logistics
  6. Environment
  7. Environmental health

D. **Coordination Priorities**

Field Reporting

Contents

Guidance Notes

Reporting can be tedious—especially when one is up at midnight struggling to organize the data and to write the report. The reporting burden can be eased by data gathering templates whose structure facilitates comprehensive and concise reporting afterward. What templates cannot provide is analytic insight. The greatest weakness in health situation reporting—whether initial REA or subsequent periodic reporting—is poor data analysis. Data regurgitation from secondary sources without analysis is rampant. Data and context analysis explain what has occurred, why it has occurred, and what is likely to occur in the future. Field grade insight with cost-effective recommendations are the hallmarks of competent medical coordinators.

Rapid Epidemiological Assessment Report (Document 5.1)
Document 5.1 derives from two Documents already discussed—Document "Rapid Epidemiological Assessment", Chapter 3, REA I–XII and Document "Rapid Epidemiological Assessment Recommendations", Chapter 4, REA Recommendations XIII). Together, items I–XIII comprise the bulk of the report. Two additional parts are needed—Executive Summary at the beginning of the report, and Documentation Annexes at the end of the report.

If the REA Report is written from scratch using the documents provided, the report may be generated in about a day. If the REA Report is drafted progressively as data are produced by the REA process, the report may be completed in several hours. Under that circumstance, the rate-limiting step in report writing is the documentation annexes.

Weekly Health Situation Report (Document 5.2)
Health Situation Report is generally produced weekly in the acute disaster setting. It focuses on updates and new findings. It is often viewed as a compliance burden which most agencies attempt to remedy through a short template. However, a sitrep is also a leadership opportunity to analyze the field, and its template is typically not granular enough. Document 5.2 is very detailed—7 pages in length. The content details are not intended to be prescriptive, but rather probative in coherent ways. A sitrep can be written in about an hour. The main headings recur week-to-week, and the sub-headings serve as prompts for discussion. If no new details emerge that week, then that part of the report is summarized as "nothing new" or suppressed altogether.

© David A. Bradt 2019
D. A. Bradt, C. M. Drummond, *Reference Manual for Humanitarian Health Professionals*,
https://doi.org/10.1007/978-3-319-69871-7_5

Health Sector Status Summary (Document 5.3) [1]

Health sector status summary concisely tabulates the subsector lead agency, milestones and benchmarks, current status, and overall priority/unmet need. This summary, unlike other documents, requires input from outside agencies. It is a conceptual burden to succinctly profile the current status of an entire evolving disaster outside of the scope of one's organization, and for that reason, the task is commonly avoided. However, failing to do so misses a threefold opportunity:

1. the leadership opportunity to quickly demonstrate an ability to organize cross-cutting information relevant to numerous stakeholders in the disaster response;
2. the strategic opportunity to shape the optics of disaster relief by proper prioritization of relief issues;
3. the tactical opportunity to quickly orient new staff to the field.

All opportunities enable the medical coordinator to contribute to a common understanding of disaster issues in the field and should not be overlooked. An example from the field may be found in *Prehospital and Disaster Medicine* [2].

References

1. Bradt, D. A., Drummond, C. M. (2003). From complex emergencies to terrorism—new tools for health sector coordination in conflict-associated disasters. *Prehospital and Disaster Medicine, 18*(3), 263–271.
2. Bradt, D. A. (2009). Evidence-based decision-making (part 2): applications in disaster relief operations. *Prehospital and Disaster Medicine, 24*(6), 479–492.

Document 5.1
RAPID EPIDEMIOLOGICAL ASSESSMENT REPORT
Date

EXECUTIVE SUMMARY

    A.   **Introduction** (copied from REA I A–B)

    B.   **REA Principal Findings and Analysis** (copied from REA XII)

    C.   **Recommendations** (copied from REA XIII)

I.   INTRODUCTION

    A.   **Hazard History Abridged**

    B.   **Current Disaster**

    C.   **Immediate Response of Host Government Authorities**

    D.   **Your Mission**

II.   SOURCES AND METHODS

    A.   **Assessment Team Composition**

    B.   **Assessment Area and Dates**

    C.   **Information Sources and Assessment Methods**

    D.   **Logistics of Assessment Team**

    E.   **Constraints**

III.   PRE-EXISTING INDICATORS (summarize Tool 3.T1)

IV.   DISASTER IMPACT

    A.   **Area Affected** (focus on most affected)

    B.   **Population Affected** (focus on most affected; see Tool 3.T2a, 3.T2b)

    C.   **Damage Assessment** (focus on most affected area; see Tool 3.T2c)

    D.   **Secondary Disasters and Threats**

    E.   **Disaster Impact Summary**

V.   CURRENT EPIDEMIOLOGICAL INDICATORS

    A.   **Epidemiology**

    B.   **Outbreaks and Epidemics**

    C.   **Epidemiological Summary**

VI.   HEALTH SECTOR FUNCTIONAL STATUS

    A.   **Public Health Services** (focus on service disruptions, adequacy)

        1.   Data

        2.   Issues summary

    B.   **Health Facilities and Clinical Services** (focus on service disruptions, adequacy; see Tool 3.T2c)

        1.   Data
        2.   Issues summary

    C.   **Human Resources** (focus on catchment area of interest)

        1.   Data
        2.   Issues summary

    D.   **Essential Medical Products and Technologies**

        1.   Data
        2.   Issues summary

    E.   **Health Information Systems**

        1.   Data
        2.   Issues summary

    F.   **Health Financing** (disaster-specific)

        1.   Data
        2.   Issues summary

    G.   **Health Leadership and Governance**

        1.   Data
        2.   Issues summary

    H.   **Health Sector Functional Status Summary**

VII. OTHER SECTORS

    A.   **Security**

        1.   Data
        2.   Issues summary

    B.   **Protection** (who, where, from what)

        1.   Data
        2.   Issues summary

    C.   **Safety** (for all parties to relief operation)

        1.   Data
        2.   Issues summary

    D.   **Search and Rescue** (if ongoing)

        1.   Data
        2.   Issues summary

    E.   **Logistics** (esp for relief agencies)

        1.   Data
        2.   Issues summary

    F.   **Environment**

        1.   Data
        2.   Issues summary

G.   **Environmental Health**

    1.   Data

    2.   Issues summary

VIII. RESPONSE OF DOMESTIC (HOST COUNTRY) AUTHORITIES

A.   **Disaster Management Mechanism**

B.   **Emergency Protection Powers in Disasters**

C.   **Advisories and Decrees**

D.   **Issues Summary**

IX. RESPONSE OF INTERNATIONAL COMMUNITY

A.   **Coordination of International Assistance**

B.   **Intervenors**

C.   **Multi-party Assessments**

D.   **International Appeals**

E.   **Issues Summary**

X. RESPONSE OF REPORTING AGENCY

A.   **Assessment Activities Undertaken**

B.   **Assistance Projects/Activities Undertaken**

C.   **Coordination of External Assistance**

D.   **Collaboration in Partnership Development**

E.   **Support to Civil Society**

F.   **Transition to Early Recovery**

G.   **Issues Summary**

XI. OPERATIONAL CONSTRAINTS

A.   **Security**

B.   **Political/Administrative**

C.   **Logistical**

D.   **Technical**

E.   **Economic**

F.   **Developmental**

XII. REA PRINCIPAL FINDINGS AND ANALYSIS (list major findings from section summaries; emphasize summaries bolded below as most relevant to health sector; use phrases, not sentences)

A.   **Disaster Impact Summary** (see REA IV E)

B.   **Epidemiological Summary** (see REA V C)

C. **Health Sector Functional Status Summary** (see REA VI H)

D. Security, Protection, and Safety (see REA VII A, B, C)

E. Search and Rescue (see REA VII D)

F. Logistics (see REA VII E)

G. Environment (see REA VII F)

H. **Environmental Health** (see REA VII G)

I. **Stated Needs of Health Authorities** (see REA VIII A10)

J. **Major Gaps** (see REA IX E)

K. **Operational Constraints** (see REA XI)

L. Duration of Emergency Phase (see REA VIII C1)

M. Future Risk Factors (see REA IV D)

XIII. RECOMMENDATIONS

A. **Information Priorities**

B. **Health Intervention Priorities**

C. **Other Sectoral Intervention Priorities**

D. **Coordination Priorities**

E. Program Implementation

XIV. DOCUMENTATION ANNEXES

A. **Terms of Reference**

B. **List of Team Members** (name, role, deployment location, time period)

C. **List of Contacts** (name, title, location)

D. **Itinerary and Chronology** (meetings, site visits)

E. **Records and Reports**

F. **Surveys and Surveillance**

G. **Testimonies**

H. **Photographs and Maps**

I. **Other Primary and Secondary Source Documents**

J. **Technical Notes**

K. **Glossary** (may place at beginning of report after Executive Summary)

Document 5.2
WEEKLY HEALTH SITUATION REPORT
Date

I. **SITUATION ON ARRIVAL** (first report only)

  A. **Disaster Impact** (see REA IV)

II. **CURRENT HEALTH INDICATORS**

  A. **Population Affected**

    1. Census
    2. Location
    3. Population movements

  B. **Disease Surveillance Reporting**

    1. Data sources
      a. report forms per …
      b. case definitions per …
    2. Collection interval

  C. **Epidemiology** (structure per REA V A)

    1. Mortality
      a. total deaths, excess mortality
      b. proportional mortality
        (1) cause-specific proportion of D_T (diarrhea, measles have each caused up to 40% of D_T in acute emergencies)
        (2) D_T/P_T % (if $D_T \geq 1\%$ of P_T)
      c. death rates and trends
        (1) crude (< 1/10,000/d; > 2 is critical)
        (2) age-specific e.g., 0–5 DR (< 2/10,000/d; > 4 is critical) (often 50% of D_T)
        (3) disease-specific (uncommonly used)
        (4) excess (crisis death rate—baseline death rate)
      d. case-fatality ratios
        (1) diarrhea (cholera 2–50%, dysentery 2–20%; target is CFR < 1%)
        (2) ARI (pneumonia 2–20%)
        (3) malaria
        (4) measles (2–30%)
        (5) malnutrition (associated with 50% of U5 deaths)
        (6) trauma (20% of civilian injured in acute military conflict)
    2. Morbidity
      a. total cases
      b. proportional morbidity
        (1) acute disease (epi estimates underlying early versions of EHKs)
          (a) adult presentations (1 adult obtains ~4 consults/yr; 5000 adults obtain ~5000 consults/3 mo) % adults presenting with: GI 25%, ARI 20%, MS 15%, GU 15%, malaria 10%, trauma 5%, anemia 5%, ocular 5%
          (b) pedes (1 child obtains ~5 consults/yr; 5000 children obtain ~6500 consults/3 mo) % pedes presenting with: GI 30%, ARI 30%, worms 20%, malaria 15%, trauma 10%, anemia 10%, ocular 10%, otic 5%
        (2) chronic disease (20% of P_T)

c. incidence rates and trends
  (1) presentation rate/d (1% baseline-10% in CDs)
  (2) age-specific (high risk = U5, O50)
  (3) disease-specific
    (a) diarrhea (AR 50%/mo in U5 excluding below)
      (i) dysentery (AR 5–30% over 1–3 mo in P_T)
      (ii) cholera (AR 1–5% over 1–4 mo in P_T)
    (b) ARI (AR 50%/mo in U5 esp in cold weather)
    (c) malaria (AR 50%/mo in P_T non-immune; 2%/mo in P_T immune (WHO))
      holo-endemic—intense transmission year-round (Congo)
      (6–10 infections/child/yr; mortality highest in U5 and preg F)
      hyper-endemic—intense transmission seasonally (W. Afr) (4–6 infections/child/yr; mortality across all ages)
      hypo-endemic—low transmission year-round (Thai-Burma) (1 infection/person/yr; mortality across all ages)
    (d) measles (AR 10%/epidemic in U12 non-immunized; 10–75% of cases have complications depending on health status)
    (e) malnutrition
      (i) macro (PEM 10% with $Z < -2$, 1% with $Z < -3$)
      (ii) micro (vitamins A–D; Fe, I)
    (f) trauma
      (i) (para)military conflict
      (ii) rape
      (iii) domestic violence
      (iv) motor vehicle trauma
    (g) mental health
      (i) adjustment disorders (debilitating grief reactions)
      (ii) psychiatric disease
      (iii) violence
      (iv) drug abuse

D. **Outbreaks and Epidemics** (structure per REA V B, or update since last report)
  1. Recent or ongoing
    a. etiology
    b. date of first case(s)
    c. location
    d. number of cases or attack rate
    e. consequences or current status
  2. Potential
    a. wide geographic relevance
      (1) measles
      (2) cholera (dehydrating diarrhea)
      (3) shigella (bloody diarrhea)
      (4) meningococcus (meningitis)
      (5) hepatitis A, E (acute jaundice syndrome)
      (6) influenza
    b. specific geographic relevance
      (1) malaria
      (2) viral hemorrhagic fevers (e.g., yellow fever, lassa fever, dengue HF)
      (3) typhoid (FUO)
      (4) leishmaniasis
      (5) polio
      (6) other (e.g., typhus, plague)

       c.   specific age groups
          (1)   polio (acute flaccid paralysis)
          (2)   neonatal tetanus

   E.   **Epidemiological Summary**

III.   HEALTH SECTOR FUNCTIONAL STATUS (structure per REA VI, or update since last report)

   A.   **Public Health Services** (focus on service disruptions, adequacy)

      1.   Disease prevention
         a.   primary prevention
           (1)   measles vaccination
           (2)   EPI restart
           (3)   other epidemic diseases
         b.   communicable disease control programs
           (1)   diarrhea
           (2)   ARI
           (3)   malaria
           (4)   HIV
           (5)   TB
           (6)   other
      2.   Epidemiological surveillance system
         a.   system objectives
         b.   health events/indicator conditions and case definitions
         c.   system components and flow chart of operations
         d.   level of usefulness
         e.   system attributes
         f.   system resource requirements
      3.   Epidemic preparedness and response
         a.   plan of action and coordinating committee
           (1)   public health incident command system (PHICS)
           (2)   cholera command and control center (C4)
         b.   clinical case definitions
         c.   case mgmt guidelines for communicable diseases with epidemic potential
         d.   outbreak mgmt protocol
           (1)   surveillance definitions
           (2)   alert thresholds
           (3)   rapid response teams to investigate case reports
           (4)   epidemic investigation kits to use
           (5)   specimens to collect
           (6)   labs to verify diagnosis (including sample sharing for confirmatory testing)
           (7)   patients to identify, isolate, and treat (inpatient and outpatient settings)
               (a)   isolation areas to organize
               (b)   treatments to plan
           (8)   contacts to trace and ? quarantine
           (9)   hotlines to use for notifiable diseases and rumor investigation
         e.   primary and secondary prevention
           (1)   infection control protocols
           (2)   commodities
               (a)   vaccines (e.g., measles, meningitis)
               (b)   drugs (e.g., prophylactic meds)
               (c)   chemicals (e.g., soap, Ca hypochlorite)
               (d)   supplies (e.g., chlorimetric and colimetric monitors)
               (e)   equipment (e.g., PPE)

        f.   resource prepositioning (stockpiles, supply chain)

        g.   information mgmt and crisis communication (media strategy)

           (1) health authorities, WHO

           (2) political authorities

           (3) community leaders and public

               (a)   social mobilization

               (b)   hygiene promotion and health education

               (c)   behavioral change communication (BCC)

        h.   contingency planning for epidemic consequences (ref DHHS flu pandemic plan)

           (1) provision of essential services (lifelines)

           (2) corpse mgmt

    4.   Health promotion (relevant to disaster response)

        a.   targeted diseases

           (1) acute epidemic diseases

           (2) chronic diseases—HTN, DM, HIV/TB, asthma

        b.   health promotion activities

           (1) community health education

           (2) provider education

    5.   Health protection (relevant to disaster response)

        a.   air quality (e.g., wildfires, volcanic eruptions)

        b.   injury control

        c.   occupational health and safety

        d.   hazardous materials (e.g., chemical releases)

        e.   disaster risk reduction (e.g., safe hospitals)

B.   **Health Facilities and Clinical Services** (focus on service disruptions, adequacy)

	Mobile Clinics	Fixed Clinics	Health Centers	District Hospitals
1. Health facilities				
2. Clinical services				
3. Special services				
a. child health				
b. reproductive health				
c. trauma				
d. mental health				
e. chronic diseases				
4. Case management				
5. Infection control				

C.   **Human Resources**

    1.   Additions and subtractions since last report

D.   **Essential Medical Products and Technologies** (status, new issues)

E.   **Health Information Systems** (status, new issues)

F.   **Health Financing** (status, new issues)

G.   **Health Leadership and Governance** (status, new issues)

IV.   **OTHER SECTORS** (structure per REA VII, or update since last report)

A.   **Security**

B.   **Protection** (who, where, from what)

C.   **Safety** (for all parties to relief operation)

D.   **Search and Rescue** (if relevant to relief operation)

E.   **Logistics**

    F.   **Environment**

    G.   **Environmental Health**

V.   RESPONSE OF DOMESTIC (HOST COUNTRY) AUTHORITIES

    A.   **Key Decisions and Actions**

    B.   **Adequacy of Coordination**

VI.   RESPONSE OF INTERNATIONAL COMMUNITY

    A.   **Updates from HC, HCT, ICCG**

    B.   **Status of Appeals**

    C.   **New Actors**

VII.   RESPONSE OF REPORTING AGENCY—PROGRAM IMPLEMENTATION

    A.   **Brief Analysis of External Situation**

    B.   **Project-specific Outputs**

        1.   Direct services to beneficiaries
        2.   Indirect services to beneficiaries
            a.   Rapid epidemiological assessment
            b.   Inter-agency medical coordination
            c.   Standardized case management
            d.   Environmental health
            e.   Epidemic preparedness and response
            f.   Disease surveillance
            g.   Special surveys
            h.   Health policy and personnel planning
            i.   Immunization programs
            j.   Medical logistics
            k.   Hazard specific issues
        3.   Capacity building

    C.   **Resource Management**

        1.   Human resources
            a.   team structure and function
            b.   staff presence (quantify)
                (1) R&R schedules
                (2) incoming briefings
                (3) end-of-mission debriefings
            c.   upcoming staff selection
                (1) internationals
                (2) local staff
            d.   major gaps
        2.   Material resources
            a.   major gaps
        3.   Financial resources
            a.   major gaps
        4.   Donations
            a.   Medical consumables
            b.   IT
            c.   Other in-kind

D.   **New Assessments**

E.   **Operational Constraints**

    1.   Security
    2.   Political/Administrative
    3.   Logistical (operational support)
        a.   comms
        b.   transport
        c.   office set-up
        d.   food and lodging
    4.   Technical
    5.   Economic
    6.   Developmental

F.   **VIP Visitors**

G.   **Team Safety and Health**

    1.   Safety and security plan
        a.   SOPs
            (1)   activities of daily living
            (2)   warden system
            (3)   vehicle safety
            (4)   office safety
            (5)   residential safety
    2.   Communications plan
    3.   Staff health emergency plan
        a.   staff health records
        b.   prophylaxis (e.g., malaria)
        c.   field medical care
        d.   medevac
    4.   Contingency plans
        a.   fire
        b.   individual adverse events (kidnapping, carjacking)
        c.   security instability (e.g., insurgent attack)
        d.   team evacuation plan

H.   **Meetings Held**

I.   **Work Products Produced**

J.   **Leadership Opportunities**

K.   **Upcoming Deadlines and Explosive Issues**

VIII. FUTURE PLANS / NEXT STEPS

A.   **Information Needs**

B.   **Intervention Plans**

C.   **Inputs Required**

    1.   Staff (position, where, when, TOR)
    2.   Material
    3.   Financial

D.   **Follow-up**

Document 5.3
HEALTH SECTOR STATUS SUMMARY

Site: _____   Date: _____

Components of Assistance	Milestones and Benchmarks	Status	Priority	Lead/Contact
	Rapid Epidemiological Assessment and Monitoring			
Security	Humanitarian space accessible			
Communication	Radio handset provision			
Transport	Vehicles available, suitable for terrain			
Beneficiary identification and access	Site mapping			
	Registration			
Rapid epidemiological assessment	Template			
Assessment priorities	Population size, vulnerability, M & M			
	Public Health and Clinical Services			
Immunization	Measles coverage rate			
	Vitamin A distribution			
Clinical services	Complete camp/site allocation			
PHC	Service delivery			
Mobile clinics	Service delivery			
Hospitals	Service delivery			
Standardized case management	Clinical case definitions			
	Treatment protocols			
	Essential drugs			
	Referral guidelines			
	Secondary prevention measures			
Special needs				
Reproductive health	Service delivery—MISP, SGBV			
Maternal-child health	Service delivery			
Mental health	Service delivery			
HIV/AIDS	Service delivery—VCT, PMTCT, SCM			
Trauma care	Service delivery—EMS to rehab			
Epidemic preparedness				
Comm. diseases of epidemic potential	Clinical case definitions			
	Case management guidelines			
Outbreak management protocol	Rapid response team to investigate			
	Specimen collection protocol to follow			
	Reference lab to identify			
	Patients to isolate			
	Contact tracing			

Communicable disease control					
EPI	National program				
Malaria	National program				
TB/HIV	National program				
Community Health Education	Culturally appropriate messages				
Quality improvement	Site monitoring visits				
Epidemiological Surveillance					
Data source identification	Reporting sites				
Data management	Routine epi data flow				
	Data collection and analysis				
	Reporting and dissemination				
Special surveys	Methodology				
Environmental Health Services					
Water supply	Minimum standards				
Food supply	Minimum standards				
Supplementary feeding	Minimum standards				
Sanitation	Minimum standards				
Shelter	Minimum standards				
Vector control	Service delivery				
Health Sector Coordination					
Inventory of organizations	Contact list				
Cluster/sectoral coordination meetings	Schedule				
Health system catchments	Defined				
Agency area-specific task designations	Operational mapping with PHA/DHA				
Health personnel/team credentialing	Defined process				
Drug importation/medical logistics	Defined process				
Provincial health authority capacity bldg	Self-sufficient health sector mgmt				
Contingency planning	Plan developed and disseminated				

Compiled: _____

Source: adapted from D Bradt, C Drummond in *Prehospital and Disaster Medicine* © 2003. Used with permission.

Field Project and Staff Management

Contents

Guidance Notes

This section addresses project and staff management. It cannot do complete justice to the complexity of these two important functions. However, it is informed by our failures in managing them. The Documents in this section focus, therefore, on prevention—how to prevent showstoppers before they undermine field projects and staff.

Project Planning Overview (Document 6.1)

Project planning is complicated. Document 6.1 gives an overview. Before going to the field, it is helpful to be familiar with planning precursors such as context analysis, stakeholder analysis, SWOT analysis, and force field analysis. It is also helpful to be familiar with planning tools such as problem trees, objectives trees, project maps, logframes, and workplans. There is a fair amount of homework to do. Clear and concise overviews of project planning exist in the bibliography of many relief organizations. One of the best is "Project Development—From Problem Identification to Final Proposal", unpublished but available through WHO Emergency Operations in Geneva. Certain planning steps have particular boundary conditions or sensitivities for an organization. Director's input is especially important in establishing priorities, selecting a strategy, and developing a budget. Director's input can also help unmask incompatible specifications in a proposal that one unwittingly tries to satisfy. Management guru Peter Drucker considers this situation the most dangerous for a manager.

Project Plan of Action (Document 6.2)

Document 6.2 is an outline for a project plan of action. It may be useful when your organization does not stipulate one. Tools 6.1–6.3 may assist the planning process at tabletop discussions in the field. The use of a logframe may not improve the quality of services described in a proposal. However, it will improve funding prospects with a serious donor.

Health personnel tend to focus on the service end of a project rather than the procurement end. They should pay attention to medical logistics. Amateurs discuss strategy, but professionals discuss logistics.

Tool 6.T4 may be useful for abstracting project details prior to embarking on monitoring and evaluation visits. Tool 6.T5 may be useful when considering remote management.

© David A. Bradt 2019
D. A. Bradt, C. M. Drummond, *Reference Manual for Humanitarian Health Professionals*,
https://doi.org/10.1007/978-3-319-69871-7_6

Disaster Medicine Staff Qualifications (Tool 6.T6) [1]

Health care providers play key roles in many disaster relief operations. Epidemiological justifications exist for clinical skills in pediatrics, obstetrics, emergency medicine, internal medicine, infectious diseases, tropical medicine, surgery, rehabilitation medicine, and psychiatry. Unfortunately, clinicians from donor countries practicing in international settings tend to have inflated notions of their own importance. Field conditions with limited resources place predictable constraints on specialist clinicians. These constraints include being western trained, hospital-based, technology dependent, procedurally oriented, invasive, monolingual, and hazard naïve. Multi-disciplinary generalists generally prove to be more useful.

Staff selection is a critical and under-examined issue in disaster management. Medical coordinators are frequently called upon to advise or approve the selection of health personnel for their teams. This action requires understanding multiple dimensions of performance in disaster medicine. Tool 6.T6 provides a quantitative approach to assessing the criterion-referenced qualifications. This schema identifies benchmarks for health technical qualifications, field experience, language competence, and peer awards. The process is highly specific—it limits false positive errors of commission in personnel selection albeit at risk of false negative errors of omission. Between 25–50% level of qualification, we generally consider candidates suitable for domestic deployment as disaster medical officers. Between 50–75% level of qualification, we generally consider candidates suitable for international deployment as disaster medical officers. Over 75% level of qualification, we generally consider candidates suitable for international deployment as disaster medical coordinators. Additional exploration of criterion-referenced qualifications in disaster medicine appears in *Prehospital and Disaster Medicine* [1].

Staff selection is the beginning of human resource management responsibilities for medical coordinators. Briefing, tasking, supervising, updating, evaluating, debriefing, and discharging staff are all additional important duties. The Situational Leadership® model of Hersey [2] and Blanchard [3] has a lot to offer the medical coordinator along with guidance on its one minute implementation. By far, the most challenging aspect in human resources is managing incompetent or unruly staff—particularly those with passive-aggressive personalities, substance abuse, or security neglect. This aspect of management is woefully addressed by many organizations which thereby endanger their programs, their beneficiaries, as well as their staff. Medical coordinators must recognize an untenable position when they are hired with the responsibility, but without the authority, to fulfill their management duties. Accessible advice and ongoing support from their human resources department are critical.

References

1. Bradt, D. A., Drummond, C. M. (2007). Professionalization of disaster medicine—an appraisal of criterion-referenced qualifications. *Prehospital and Disaster Medicine, 22*(5), 360–368.
2. Hersey P. Situational leadership model. Available from https://situational.com/the-cls-difference/situational-leadership-what-we-do/.
3. Blanchard, K. H., Zigarmi, P., Zigarmi, D. (1985). *Leadership and the one minute manager*. New York: Morrow.

Document 6.1
PROJECT PLANNING OVERVIEW

Disaster Planning Types

1. Strategic
2. Preparedness
3. Operations
   a. Security
   b. Communications
   c. Transport
   d. Staff health
   e. Beneficiary programs
4. Contingency
5. Evaluation

Planning precursors

1. Situation/Context Analysis
2. Stakeholder Analysis—identify stakeholders, capacity, and vulnerability for all areas of the potential work environment
3. SWOT Analysis—strengths, weaknesses, opportunities, and threats
4. Force Field Analysis—forces at play
5. Director's Vision of Success*—how you know when you get there
   a. mission and goal(s)
   b. boundary conditions—consequences to be avoided

Planning steps

1. Priorities*
2. Assumptions and Constraints
3. Problem Tree—performs root cause analysis, then summarizes cause and effects in a problem tree
4. Objectives Tree—reformulates problems identified above into objectives that are desirable and achievable, then summarizes means and ends in an objectives tree
5. Feasibility Analysis—technical, administrative, political, economic, and developmental analysis; analysis of alternatives; impact analysis (positive and negative); strategy selection*
6. Project Map—shows hierarchal relationship between purpose, components, results, and activities
7. Logframe—summarizes how and why
8. Workplan (implementation schedule, resource schedule)—summarizes when, and with what resources
9. Cost Schedule* (budget)—summarizes planned expenditures
10. Monitoring and Evaluation Plan
11. Reports Schedule
12. SOPs
13. Contingency Plans

* items need director's guidance/feedback

Document 6.2
PROJECT PLAN OF ACTION
Date

Executive Summary

    A. **Goals** (Agency Intent)

    B. **Strategy, Objectives, and Expected Results**

I.   SITUATION/CONTEXT ANALYSIS

    A. **Disaster History**

    B. **Sociopolitical and Cultural Context** (on health status, health care services, and interventions)

    C. **Security Situation**

    D. **Resources and Capacities Available**

    E. **Roles and Influence of Major Stakeholders** (e.g., military, non-state actors)

    F. **Health Services** (SWOT and Constraints)

    G. **Disaster Expected Evolution** (lessons learned from past experience)

    H. **Reason for Agency Assistance**

II.   GOALS (Agency Priorities and Intent)

    A. **Mission**

        1. Goals
        2. Beneficiaries
        3. Geographic location
        4. Timeframe

    B. **Vision of End State**

    C. **Boundary Conditions**

        1. Key decisions
        2. Antigoals (unwanted outcomes)

III.   ASSUMPTIONS AND CONSTRAINTS

    A. **Assumptions**

        1. Security and socioeconomic assumptions
        2. Epidemiological assumptions
        3. Health resource assumptions
        4. Donor assumptions

    B. **Constraints**

IV. STRATEGY, OBJECTIVES, AND EXPECTED RESULTS

A. Principles

1. Comprehensive approach involving PPRR
   a. all-hazards
   b. human and animal health
2. Integrated approach involving prepared community
3. Build on existing platforms and investments
4. Coordinate and leverage resources with other donors and private sector
5. Focus on high yield activities in high risk areas

B. Strategy

1. Population targeted
2. Subsector goods and services provided
3. Health system levels of care supported/restored

C. Objectives (e.g., in communicable diseases)

1. Prepare for epidemics
2. Prevent and control vaccine-preventable illnesses
3. Prevent and control vector-borne illnesses
4. Intensify disease surveillance system

D. Expected Results

1. 80% of targeted population or facilities

V. KEY ACTIVITIES AND PERFORMANCE INDICATORS (Logframe or Plan of Action by Objective)

Activity	Indicators	Means of Verification	Verifier	Input Needed	Date Done
Objective 1					
Activity 1	•	•			
Activity 2	•	•			
Activity 3	•	•			
Objective 2					
Activity 1	•	•			
Activity 2	•	•			
Activity 3	•	•			
Objective 3					
Activity 1	•	•			
Activity 2	•	•			
Activity 3	•	•			
Objective 4					
Activity 1	•	•			
Activity 2	•	•			
Activity 3	•	•			

VI. PROGRAM DESCRIPTION

    A. **Implementation Plan**

    B. **Monitoring and Evaluation**

    C. **Transition or Exit Strategy**

VII. OUTPUTS AND OUTCOMES

    A. **Outputs**

    B. **Impacts and Outcomes**

        1. Environmental
        2. Health
        3. Socioeconomic
        4. Political
        5. Financial

    C. **Sustainability**

    D. **Contingency Planning**

VIII. ACTIVITY OVERSIGHT

    A. **Organization Executive Officers**

    B. **Project External Advisory Panel**

    C. **Project Leadership Team**

    D. **Field Supervisors**

    E. **Field Staff**

IX. REPORTING

    A. **Resource Management**

        1. Human resources
        2. Material resources
        3. Financial resources

    B. **Other POA Deliverables**
        1. Operations research

    C. **Incident Reports**

    D. **Unexpected Consequences**

X. SCHEDULE (GANTT TABLE)

XI. BUDGET

XII. ABBREVIATIONS

XIII.   **TECHNICAL ANNEXES** (in chronological order of development)

    A.   **Situation/Context Analysis**

        1.   Stakeholder analysis (organization, community, population)
            a.   identification
            b.   strengths and weaknesses
            c.   implementation capacity
            d.   vulnerability
            e.   preparatory assistance needed
            f.   linkages
        2.   SWOT analysis (strengths & weaknesses of your org; opportunities and threats of the environment)
        3.   Force field analysis (forces at play)

    B.   **Goals** (Agency Priorities and Intent)

    C.   **Assumptions and Constraints**

    D.   **Problem Tree** (root cause analysis)

    E.   **Objectives Tree** (means to ends)

    F.   **Feasibility Analysis**

        1.   Technical
        2.   Administrative
        3.   Political
        4.   Economic
        5.   Developmental
        6.   Impact (positive and negative)

    G.   **Project Map**

    H.   **Logframe**

    I.   **Workplan**

        1.   Implementation schedule
        2.   Resource schedule

    J.   **Cost Schedule** (budget)

    K.   **Monitoring and Evaluation Plan**

    L.   **Reports Schedule** (templates)

    M.   **SOPs** (if not covered by the safety and security plan)

    N.   **Contingency Plans**

        1.   Major staff sickness (e.g., pandemic flu)
        2.   Border shutdown

Tool 6.T1
PROJECT MAP

Project Objective, Components 1–2

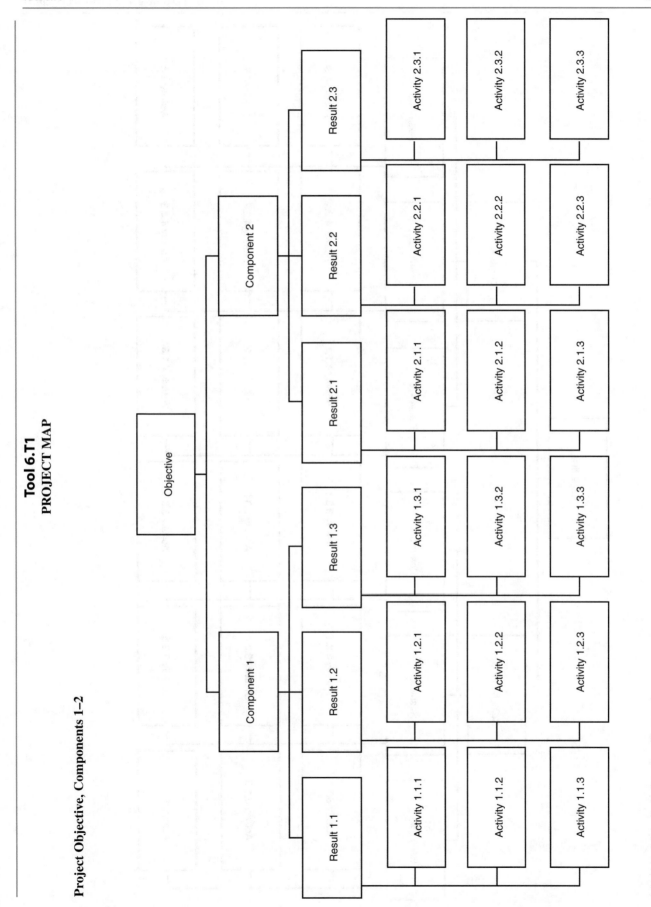

Project Objective, Components 3–4

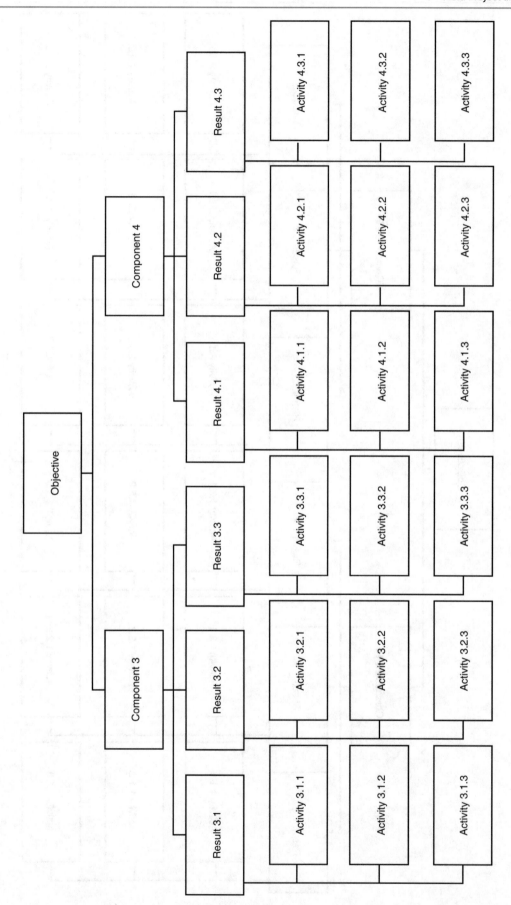

Tool 6.T2
LOGICAL FRAMEWORK DEFINITIONS AND PROCESS

logical framework approach—analytical, presentational, and management tool involving a four part process which culminates in the logical framework matrix (logframe)

- problem analysis
- stakeholder analysis
- objectives analysis
- options analysis

The process serves to:

- analyze the existing situation
- identify vested interests (pro and con)
- establish a logical hierarchy of means by which objectives will be reached
- identify potential risks
- establish how outputs and outcomes might best be monitored
- present a project summary in standard format

logical framework matrix (logframe)—product of the logical framework approach

- **goal**—sectoral or national development impact to which the project contributes (written in the infinitive)
- **objective/purpose**—developmental outcome expected at the end of the project to which all components contribute (written in the infinitive)
- **component of objective**—specific outcome of each project output/activity area achieved by delivering specific outputs (written in the infinitive); each component has its specific sectoral, institutional, or technical focus and is likely to be managed by different groups within the targeted institution
  - training program design and delivery
  - facilities upgrading
  - project management
- **results/outputs**—direct measurable results in goods and services of the project (written in future perfect e.g., something will have been produced)
- **activities**—tasks carried out to deliver the identified outputs (written in present tense)
- **indicators**—measures of progress toward project goal, measure of extent to which component objectives have been achieved, quantity and quality of outputs, timing of delivery; they are SMART
  - specific
  - measurable
  - achievable (under one's responsibility, authority, influence, and technical competence)
  - relevant
  - time-bound
- **means of verification (MOVs)**
  - who will collect data
  - what source, where located
  - when and how often
  - how to collect the data
  - what format to record the data
- **assumptions**—future conditions affecting project success over which the project manager has no direct control e.g., price stabilization, rainfall, land reform, etc.
  - assumption—a condition, stated positively, upon which the project is dependent for objectives to be achieved
  - risk—a condition, stated negatively, which may prevent objectives from being achieved
  - killer assumption—an assumption judged as highly likely to change and critically undermine the project; when so identified, the project ought to be abandoned or redesigned

Logframe structure and completion sequence:

Project Description	Indicators	MOVs	Assumptions
1. Goal	10. Indicators	11. MOVs	
2. Objectives	12. Indicators	13. MOVs	9. Assumptions
3. Components	14. Indicators	15. MOVs	8. Assumptions
4. Results/Outputs	16. Indicators	17. MOVs	7. Assumptions
5. Activities	milestones per activity scheduled	periodic reports	6. Assumptions

Overall, a logframe is a matrix, a logic, and a grammar. It can be cumbersome for the uninitiated. Many organizations, including WHO, use a simplified form of logframe to facilitate field use. This simplified approach may rely on predetermined indicator libraries, activity lists by subsector, and activity-based budgets. A well-developed logframe should be the STARTING point for operational planning. Inputs—resources required to undertake activities and produce outputs—are typically not specified in logframes, but are ultimately required for operational plans. Inputs commonly include:

- personnel
- information
- materials
- property, plant, and equipment
- time
- money
- organizational inputs
- complementary inputs
- unmet needs

Example:

Project Description	Indicators	MOVs	Assumptions
Goal	reduction of infant and child mortality by 30%	routine reports baseline and follow-up surveys	regarding relevance of project to program goals
Objectives	zero cases of measles in a designated 12 month period	epidemiological surveillance	regarding impact of services
Components			
Results/Outputs	80% of defined target population immunized	survey	regarding conversion of activities into results
Activities/Services	immunization program	service records	regarding conversion of resources into activities

Tool 6.T3
LOGFRAME TEMPLATE

	Intervention Logic	Objectively Verifiable Indicators of Achievement	Sources and Means of Verification	Assumptions
Program Goal	•	•	•	•
Objective or Component	•	•	•	•
Objective or Component	•	•	•	•

Objective 1		
•		
•		•
•	•	•
Expected Results		

Objective 2		
•		
•	•	•
•	•	•
Expected Results		

Objective 3		
•		
•		•
•	•	•
Expected Results		

Tool 6.T4
PROJECT MONITORING AND EVALUATION WORKSHEET

Project Name:

Lead Agency & Subs:

Location:

Donors & Funding:

Duration:

Project Purpose:

Target Groups:

Project key contacts:

-

-

-

-

Component Description:

Component/Sector	Beneficiary Population Size	Location Province/District	When Start

General Feasibility Issues Arising

Security	**Technical**
Staff	**Administrative**
Stuff	**Political**
Spending	**Economic**
	Developmental

Project Management Issues

Ref #	Components, Outputs, and Activities	Achievements by Component	Problems and Constraints	Actions Taken or Required
	Component 1			
	Output 1			
	• Activity 1			
	• Activity 2			
	• Activity 3			
	Output 2			
	• Activity 1			
	• Activity 2			
	• Activity 3			
	Output 3			
	• Activity 1			
	• Activity 2			
	• Activity 3			
	Output 4			
	• Activity 1			
	• Activity 2			

Tool 6.T5
REMOTE MANAGEMENT WORKSHEET

I. **Definition** (ICRC [1])

The withdrawal of senior international or national humanitarian managers from the location of the provision of assistance or other humanitarian action as an adaptation to insecurity or denied access
- deviation from 'normal' programming practice
- program quality and effectiveness may suffer—particularly in impartiality of beneficiary selection and accountability of results
- may entail risk transfer to local partners
- last-resort modality short of suspending operations

II. **Rationale**

A. **Key Questions** (ECHO [2])

1. Is there an access problem due to insecurity?
    a. Are there significant access issues impairing the delivery of humanitarian assistance which the implementing partner cannot resolve?
    b. In the same geographic area, is there no other humanitarian organization (eligible for ECHO funding) with the required capacity and experience willing and able to meet the desired humanitarian needs thru direct action?
    c. Does the proposed intervention undermine efforts to resolve the security/bureaucratic obstacles?
2. Does the proposed action include acceptance-building measures?
    NB Acceptance of impartial and independent humanitarian action by local government, communities, and non-state actors is the most effective way to mitigate security risks for humanitarian workers and gain access to vulnerable populations. Insightful stakeholder mapping and experienced access negotiators are keys to the process.
    a. Does the proposed action identify actors at local, provincial, or international level who can impact access in proposed geographic areas?
    b. Does the proposed action include steps to gain, regain, or maintain acceptance of neutral and independent humanitarian action?
3. Is there a direct life-saving action?
    NB In view of associated risks, remote management is only be justified when it directly saves lives or preserves crucial livelihoods. Preparedness, early recovery, R2D, and resilience actions do not qualify.
4. Can the action be implemented without risking the lives of those undertaking the work on the ground?
    NB When management staff cannot verify the quality of the intervention, transfer of risk to field staff or to another implementer is not acceptable.
    a. Implementing partner must provide clear evidence that all possible measure have been put in place to reduce the risks for local staff undertaking the action. Implementing partner must provide clear evidence that programs are designed and delivered in manner that does not negatively impact on the security of disaster-affected communities and beneficiaries.
5. What is the source of the needs assessment in a remotely managed action?
    a. Implementing partner must specify what sources of information were used to estimate needs.
    b. Data collected remotely in conflict-affected areas (thru local staff, external partners, aerial surveillance, etc.) must be verified by direct sources (IDPs, traders community representatives, etc.).
6. Are staff on the ground adequately qualified and trained to manage the action, and are the information systems in place to provide them with needed information?
    a. Management staff must always have updated information on field level implementation.
    b. Skill gaps (technical, analytic, managerial) in field staff must be identified and remedied thru training or other measures.

7. Are the monitoring arrangements adapted for remote management?

    NB   Effective monitoring requires a minimum level of face-to-face contact between managers, field staff, and beneficiaries. When managers cannot go to field sites, it may be possible for some beneficiaries to travel to a sub-office location. If that is not possible, remote managers must seek face-to-face meetings with stakeholders from affected areas (e.g., community representatives, traditional authorities, or traders).

    NB   Risks of remote management increase over time—needs assessments may be outdated; risks may be inaccurately assessed; managers may lose touch with the field situation. "The longer humanitarian organizations rely on remote management to deliver assistance…the greater the risk that aid will become less effective" [2].

    a.   Is there a mechanism of direct contact between program managers and beneficiaries or other local stakeholders?

    b.   Are third party monitors engaged? If so, they must be external to the conflict.

B.   Indirect Monitoring Methods

1. Debriefing between iNGO and local partner
2. Mobile and web-based communications technology enabling call centers to check on staff, supplies, and operations at remote sites (difficult where field comms at remote sites are not accessible, reliable, or secure)
3. Phone complaint and feedback mechanisms (allowing beneficiaries to comment on type of assistance, quality of assistance, allegations of corruption, etc.)
4. Complaint boxes
5. Broadcasts about planned activities (generally not feasible in conflicted areas)
6. Photos or videos of commodity distribution or service delivery
7. Web-based remote monitoring (via geo-tagged photos posted online or sent by email)
8. GPS shipment tracking (barcoding of shipment, scanning at dispatch and receipt)
9. Remote sensing
10. Voucher reconciliation
11. Peer monitoring (triangulation thru discussion with organizations working in the same area)
12. Third party monitoring (private firm with skilled personnel paid by implementing partner)—increasingly seen as gold standard
13. Crowd sourcing (via SMS, internet, Facebook)

References

1. Donini, A., Maxwell, D. (2013). From face-to-face to face-to-screen: Remote management, effectiveness and accountability of humanitarian action in insecure environments. *International Review of the Red Cross*, *95*(890), 383–413. doi: https://doi.org/10.1017/S1816383114000265.
2. ECHO. (2015). *ECHO's approach to remote management*. Available from http://dgecho-partners-helpdesk.eu/actions_implementation/remote_management/start.

Tool 6.T6
DISASTER MEDICINE STAFF QUALIFICATIONS
Quantitative Assessment

Name: _____

Domain	Qualification	Points	Score
Specialty-specific Competency			
Clinical medicine	specialty board certification	5 each, maximum of 10	
	specialty board eligibility	4 each, maximum of 8	
	MD, DO, MBBS or equivalent	3	
	RN, nurse clinical specialist	2 each	
	paramedic, diploma courses	1 each	
Public health	specialty board certification	5 each, maximum of 10	
	specialty board eligibility	4 each, maximum of 8	
	DrPH or equivalent	3	
	FETP, MPH, MSPH, MAE	2 each	
	diploma courses	1 each	
Disaster management	no internationally endorsed standards at present	1/quarter year, maximum of 10	
Section Total		**30 maximum**	
Language-specific Competency		**5 point foreign service scale**	
UN languages	English and French preferred	5 maximum/language	
Other languages	only germane if used by disaster affected population or host government providers	5 maximum/language	
Section Total		**20 maximum**	
Hazard & Site-Specific Competency (Field Experience)	**assignments of > 1 month by location, hazard type, and agency**		
Military medicine in combat operations		3/month of full-time field service; maximum 10/conflict	
Field assignments in disaster impact and needs assessment, disaster relief site operations, mass casualty incident management, or disaster response project management. Military active duty in peacekeeping or humanitarian assistance operations		2/month of full-time field service; maximum 5/disaster	
Field assignments in disaster preparedness, project identification, monitoring and evaluation, education, and research		1/month of full-time field service; maximum 5/country	
Section Total		**50 maximum**	

Peer Awards in Disaster-Related Activities		
Military medicine in combat operations		10/award
UN field assignments		5/award
Red Cross field assignments		5/award
Governmental organizations, military medicine in peacekeeping or humanitarian assistance operations		5/award
Non-governmental organizations		3/award
Academic and trade associations		2/award
Section Total		**20 maximum**
Grand Total		**120 maximum**

Scoring:　30–59　consider for medical officer deployment in domestic disaster
　　　　　 60–89　consider for medical officer deployment in international disaster
　　　　　 90+　　consider for medical coordinator deployment

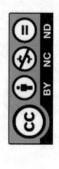

Medical Coordination

Contents

Guidance Notes

This section addresses several issues unique to medical coordinators. Medical coordinators should possess the technical competence to render an informed opinion, the administrative authority to mobilize resources, and the organizational responsibility for outcomes. Such is not always the case. If an organization is represented by someone lacking competence, authority, or responsibility, then the organization should be encouraged to send someone who has it. Health cluster coordination is the application of medical coordination skills to an interagency cluster context. This application requires specialized tools and training.

Medical Coordinator Generic Terms of Reference (Document 7.1) [1]
The Document is self-explanatory.

Medical Coordinator Work Products (Document 7.2)
Medical coordination meetings should be decisional, not just informational. Document 7.2 is a list of representative work products requiring decisions by medical coordinators. There is much overlap with the Medical Handover Checklist (Document 7.2) which evidences the match between briefing logic and field practice. Not all the work product need be produced by the medical coordinators. Some of it may exist in-country before the current disaster. However all of it will need to be applied in the context of the disaster. This documentation contributes to a reference archive critical to the effectiveness of the medical coordinator.

Health Cluster Principles of Coordination (Document 7.3)
Health Cluster Meeting Agenda (Tool 7.T1), **Meeting Process** (Tool 7.T2)
It is essential that host health authorities lead the process, and that it embraces local providers and NGOs. Local culture, practices, and beliefs must inform decisions made about health programs. One must beware of the insidious cycle of foreign

© David A. Bradt 2019
D. A. Bradt, C. M. Drummond, *Reference Manual for Humanitarian Health Professionals*,
https://doi.org/10.1007/978-3-319-69871-7_7

actors paid by foreign donors who intervene on behalf of foreign constituencies, and then use external criteria to judge the adequacy of their work.

Medical coordination meetings are an opportunity for the Ministry of Health and medical coordinators to develop consensus on health sector priorities, practices, and accountability. Meeting agenda and process are characterized in Tools 7.T1 and 7.T2. At those meetings, principles of engagement are an excellent way to begin substantive discussions. These principles typically acknowledge humanitarian values, group commitment to international best practices, and ascendancy of the host country. An example is presented in Document 7.3. The document specifics are less important in many ways than the process of developing a consensus around them. The process evidences the ability of medical coordinators to develop a consensus on non-controversial areas. A fundamental problem in health sector coordination occurs when medical coordinators cannot reach consensus early in a relief operation. This failure augurs poorly for the group's ability to develop consensus around controversial issues later in the relief effort.

Reference

1. Bradt, D. A., & Drummond, C. M. (2003). From complex emergencies to terrorism—new tools for health sector coordination in conflict-associated disasters. *Prehospital and Disaster Medicine, 18*(3), 263–271.

Document 7.1
MEDICAL COORDINATOR GENERIC TERMS OF REFERENCE
Source: adapted from WHO job descriptions

Education and Knowledge

- Post-graduate degree in public health; preferably a degree in medicine
- Excellent knowledge of the UN and NGO humanitarian community
- Knowledge of the latest health-related technical guidelines and standards

Experience

- Field experience with international organizations including UN agencies and NGOs in emergency situations (minimum 8 yr)
- Leadership, management, and coordination experience in the 8 yr identified above.

Personal Skills

- Demonstrated ability for leadership and independent decision-making
- Demonstrated management skills
- Strong negotiation and inter-personal skills
- Willingness and ability to work in hardship environments
- Readily available for deployment in emergency situations
- Cultural and gender sensitivity
- Success in developing partnerships
- Expertise in English with proficiency in another official UN language

Terms of Reference

The incumbent will work to fulfill the organization's mission:

- Provide health leadership in emergency and crisis preparedness, response, and recovery
- Prevent and reduce excess mortality and morbidity
- Ensure evidence-based actions, gap filling, and sound coordination
- Enhance accountability, predictability, and effectiveness of humanitarian health actions

Specific actions relating to the above:

- Identify health cluster partners in the relief community
- Undertake rapid epidemiological assessment
- Plan and develop health strategy
- Apply relevant standards in health program development
- Coordinate health program implementation
- Monitor adequacy of health program implementation
- Manage and report relevant data, information, and analyses on beneficiary health status, program functioning, future beneficiary needs, and country context
- Promote common and joint system to evaluate effectiveness of health program
- Advocate and mobilize resources
- Build capacity of local/national health authorities

Document 7.2
MEDICAL COORDINATOR WORK PRODUCTS

I.   COORDINATION

A.	**List of Agencies, NGOs**	contact list
B.	**Host Health System**	organigram, description
C.	**Area-activity Table (who-what-where)**	matrix
D.	**Partnership in Health Facilities** (DHO + local NGO + iNGO)	
E.	**Coordination Meetings**	meetings calendar, minutes

II. RAPID EPIDEMIOLOGICAL ASSESSMENT

A.	**Access to Affected**	geographic mapping
B.	**Methodology**	**template**
C.	**Priority Populations** (e.g., CMR >1, size >1k)	agreement

III. MINIMUM STANDARDS

A. **Environmental Health**   **minimum standards** (Sphere)

  1. Water supply
  2. Food supply
  3. Sanitation
  4. Shelter
  5. Vector control

B. **Clinical Medicine**

  1. Delivery of health services   health systems catchments
  2. Standardization of case management
      a. case definitions   **guidelines**
      b. treatment protocols (disease specific)   **guidelines** (see EHK, ELK)
      c. essential drug lists   **national guidelines** (see EHK)
      d. uniform referral practices   process
      e. secondary prevention   guidelines

IV. EPIDEMIC PREPAREDNESS

A.	**Case Definitions**	guidelines
B.	**Case Management Guidelines for Communicable Diseases**	guidelines
C.	**Outbreak Management Protocol**	**guidelines** (see ELK)

  1. Alert thresholds   **table**
  2. Staff investigation   **forms**
  3. Specimen collection   **guidelines**
  4. Lab to culture   **table**

D.	**Sources of Relevant Vaccines**	list
E.	**Resource Prepositioning**	**cholera kits**
F.	**Public Information**	**templates**

V.   COMMUNICABLE DISEASE CONTROL

    A.   **Disease-specific**   **guidelines** (see ELK)

VI.   EPIDEMIOLOGICAL SURVEILLANCE

    A.   **Data Sources**   camp logbook
    B.   **Reporting Forms**   **reporting forms**
    C.   **Collection Methods**
    D.   **Data Analysis**
    E.   **Reporting**   **weekly reports**

VII.   HEALTH POLICY AND PERSONNEL   personnel credentialing

VIII. MEDICAL LOGISTICS   **process**

bold generally pre-existing
ELK   emergency library kit
EHK   emergency health kit

Document 7.3
HEALTH CLUSTER PRINCIPLES OF COORDINATION

1. Authority to work in [country] is conferred by the Government of [country] through the Ministry of Health.

2. [Lead agency] authority to coordinate organizations in the health sector is conferred by the Ministry of Health. [Lead agency] is requested to convene health coordination meetings to establish a periodic forum at which to discuss technical and programmatic health issues affecting NGO and UN agency delivery of health services in [country].

3. Participants agree to conform to health policies and procedures established by statute of the Government of [country] and regulation of the Ministry of Health.

4. Participants agree to support minimum standards of humanitarian assistance as disseminated by the Sphere Project.

5. Participants agree to adhere to the Code of Conduct as disseminated by the Sphere Project.

6. Participants agree to fully characterize their organization's health activities in [country] to enable development of a health intervenor database which optimizes resources by identifying service gaps and preventing duplication of services.

7. Participants agree to undertake health activities relying on organizational competence to serve local needs with [lead agency] acting to encourage and coordinate multi-party involvement.

8. Meeting agendas are intended to support and complement interactions currently underway between participants and [country] health authorities.

9. Meeting discussions are intended to be interactive, field-oriented, and practical. The approach to health issues will involve disseminating information, examining problems, appraising options, developing consensus, making decisions, and implementing remedies.

10. Meeting minutes will be written by [lead agency] and disseminated to focal points among participant organizations and [country] health authorities to evidence ongoing transparency and professionalism among colleagues in humanitarian health assistance.

Tool 7.T1
HEALTH CLUSTER MEETING AGENDA

I.   **INTRODUCTIONS**

II. **INFORMATION UPDATE**

    A.   **Health Authorities Overview**

    B.   **Cluster System Update**

    C.   **Epidemiological Surveillance**

    D.   **Sectoral Issues** (integrate with subgroup reports as subgroups are established)

        1.   Security, protection, & safety
        2.   Environmental health
        3.   Public health services
            a.   disease prevention—e.g., vaccination
            b.   epidemic preparedness and outbreak response
            c.   health promotion and protection
        4.   Health facilities and clinical services
            a.   vulnerable groups and access to care
            b.   delivery of clinical health services
        5.   Medical logistics
        6.   Health financing, cost recovery

III. **DISCUSSION**

    A.   **Domain-specific** (across multiple settings, e.g., vaccination campaign)

    B.   **Setting-specific** (across multiple sectors, e.g., staff unrest in one locality)

    C.   **Provider-specific** (problems with one agency)

IV. **ACTIVITY PLANNING AND PRIORITIZATION**

Tool 7.T2
HEALTH CLUSTER MEETING PROCESS
Initial Meeting

Distribute attendance sheet and contact list

Goal: cooperation—shared goals and information

Purpose: improve the health status of the population in [specify area]

Intro round robin:
> Name, organization (may limit to 1 spokesperson/organization)
> mandates/missions, resources/capabilities, areas of responsibility, perceived operational priorities

Discussion:
> Round robin protocol
>> Who—one representative to speak for the agency (technically qualified, administratively authorized, organizationally responsible)
>> What—situation update, urgent and important issues
> TOR for the group
> SAGs & TWiGs
> Critical issues of the day
> Future meeting schedule

Follow-up:
> Action steps
> Establish next time and place

Clerical duties
- **Collect attendance sheet and contact list**
- **Write running minutes of the meeting**
  > Attendance
  > Discussion point summary (with apologies by MC for any misunderstandings or omissions)
  >> Administrative issues
  >> Documentation distributed
  >> General health issues—prioritized for follow-up at next meeting
  > Follow-up
- **Compile draft contact list**

Tool 7.T2
HEALTH CLUSTER MEETING PROCESS
Subsequent Meetings

Distribute attendance sheet and contact list
Distribute blank gap identification forms

Goal: coordination—shared tasks; collaboration—shared resources

Purpose: improve the health status of the population in [specify area]

Intro round robin:
　　　　Name, organization (may limit to 1 spokesperson/organization if too many present)

Discussion:
　　　　TOR for the group (amend/assent)
　　　　SAGs & TWiGs
　　　　Critical issues of the day
　　　　Agenda for the meeting based upon issues and interest areas (give major headings only)
　　　　　　　　Introductions (especially for new persons)
　　　　　　　　Announcements (lead governmental authority)
　　　　　　　　Subsector updates including local epidemiology
　　　　　　　　New issues (rumors and reports)
　　　　　　　　　　　　critical issues which will explode within 24 h or require action to prevent imminent death)—
　　　　　　　　　　　　　　　develop subsector interest groups based upon recurrent issues
　　　　　　　　　　　　info gaps → arrangements for initial assessment
　　　　　　　　　　　　service gaps → gap filling, special planning
　　　　　　　　Matching stated needs to locally available resources (personnel, equipment, $)

Follow-up:
　　　　Action steps
　　　　Establish next time and place

Clerical duties
- **Collect attendance sheet, contact list, and gap identification forms**
- **Write running minutes of the meeting**
　　　　Attendance
　　　　Discussion point summary (apologies by MC for any misunderstandings or omissions)
　　　　　　　　Administrative issues
　　　　　　　　Documentation distributed
　　　　　　　　Health authority announcements
　　　　　　　　General health issues—prioritized for follow-up meeting
　　　　　　　　Subsector updates
　　　　Follow-up
- **Revise contact list**
- **Compile health sector area-activity matrix from gap identification forms**
- **Compile health sector status summary**

Technical Annexes

Contents

Guidance Notes

These annexes contain compilations of frequently used reference information. This information has helped us analyze field data, generate REA and health situation reports, and answer countless questions from our colleagues. Selected comments follow below.

© David A. Bradt 2019
D. A. Bradt, C. M. Drummond, *Reference Manual for Humanitarian Health Professionals*,
https://doi.org/10.1007/978-3-319-69871-7_8

Humanitarian Programs (Annex 8.1)

Annex 8.1 contains conceptual frameworks on global clusters, humanitarian assistance, program implementation, and early recovery.

Security Sector (Annex 8.2)

Annex 8.2 contains key definitions from the Rome Statute of the International Criminal Court.

Health Sector (Annex 8.3 with glossary)

Annex 8.3 contains a broad range of core health technical information including environmental classification of water and excreta-related diseases, disease prevention measures, water treatment end points, anthropometric classifications, micronutrient deficiency states, management of chemical weapon exposures, and epi methods.

Tropical Medicine (Annex 8.4 with glossary)

Annex 8.4 contains clinical summaries of selected tropical infectious diseases. It briefly overviews pathophysiology, differential diagnosis, and management keys. The accompanying tables provide disease-specific profiles which identify the disease vector and host, clinical presentation, diagnostic lab tests, clinical epidemiology, and therapy. Table 1 on Vector-Borne and Zoonotic Diseases is organized by vector. Table 2 on Non Vector-Borne Diseases is organized by phylogeny. For detailed information on these and other communicable diseases, please refer to references cited in Section 1.

Epidemic Preparedness and Response (Annex 8.5)

Annex 8.5 contains core principles of epidemic preparedness and response.

Communicable Disease Control (Annex 8.6 with glossary)

Annex 8.6 contains an overview of selected communicable diseases of epidemic potential whose incidence, management complexity, or mortality obliges particular attention. These diseases are: diarrhea, influenza, malaria, measles, meningitis, and viral hemorrhagic fever.

Disease profiles are structured to quickly orient field staff to key issues in:
- Pathogens
- Epidemiology
- Preventive medicine
- Epidemiological surveillance
- Clinical medicine
- Epidemic management

This overview is designed to supplement the superb communicable disease toolkits produced by the WHO Communicable Disease Working Group on Emergencies. Those published toolkits are disaster-specific and typically include the following reference information:
- Health Risks for Infectious Diseases
- Risk Factors for Outbreak in Emergency Situations
- Case Definitions for Health Events
- Suggested Alert threshold to Trigger Further Investigation
- Steps in Outbreak Management
- Outbreak Alert Form
- Case Investigation Form
- Flowchart for Laboratory Confirmation of [list disease]
- Diseases Under Surveillance which Require Laboratory Confirmation

Diagnostic Laboratory (Annex 8.7 with glossary)

Annex 8.7 contains guidance on lab specimen handling and testing.

Acronyms (Annex 8.8)

Annex 8.8 contains acronyms commonly used in disaster management and humanitarian assistance (DM/HA).

Annex 8.1
HUMANITARIAN PROGRAMS

I. HUMANITARIAN ASSISTANCE VALUES AND GOALS

A. **Core Values**

1. Humanity
2. Impartiality
3. Neutrality
4. Independence

B. **Goals**

1. Save lives
2. Alleviate suffering
3. Reduce economic and social impact of disaster
4. Maintain peace and security
5. Uphold law and order (host government)
6. Support vulnerable groups
7. Implement durable solutions (UNHCR)
   a. repatriation
   b. local integration
   c. resettlement
8. Mitigate hazards

II. GLOBAL CLUSTERS AND LEADS (IASC [1, 2])

A. **Technical Areas**

1.	Nutrition		UNICEF
2.	Health		WHO
3.	Water/sanitation		UNICEF
4.	Emergency shelter	IDPs from conflict	UNHCR
		disaster situations	IFRC
5.	Food security		WFP/FAO

B. **Cross-cutting Areas**

1.	Camp coordination	IDPs from conflict	UNHCR
		disaster situations	IOM
2.	Protection		UNHCR
3.	Early recovery		UNDP
4.	Education		UNICEF/SC

C. **Common Service Areas**

1.	Logistics	WFP
2.	Emergency telecoms	WFP

III. SECTORS AND THEMES

A. **Sectors**

1. Coordination
2. Protection and Registration

    3.   Security and Demobilization
    4.   Logistics
    5.   Site Planning
    6.   Water and Sanitation
    7.   Food Aid
    8.   Agriculture
    9.   Non-food Aid (household support)
   10.   Shelter
   11.   Health
   12.   Rehabilitation
   13.   Education and Training
   14.   Economic Recovery and Community Development
   15.   Durable Solutions

B.   Cross-cutting Themes (IASC)

    1.   Human Rights & Protection
    2.   Gender
    3.   HIV/AIDS
    4.   Environment

C.   Themes Per Donor Grants Guidelines

    1.   Artisanal Production
    2.   Capacity Building/Training
    3.   Cash Distribution
    4.   Cash for Work
    5.   Children
    6.   Conflict Resolution
    7.   Gender Relations
    8.   HIV-AIDS
    9.   Host Communities
   10.   Host Government
   11.   IDPs
   12.   Information Systems
   13.   Infrastructure Rehabilitation
   14.   Livelihoods/Income Generation
   15.   Market Rehabilitation
   16.   Micro-Finance/Micro-Credit
   17.   Nomads/Pastoralists
   18.   Protection Mainstreaming
   19.   Returnees
   20.   Slavery/Trafficking
   21.   Vouchers

IV.   RELIEF PROGRAMS

A.   Keys to Emergency Relief (M Toole, Burnet Institute, Melbourne, Australia, unpublished)

    1.   Intervene early
    2.   Support, not undermine, community coping strategies
    3.   Prevent communities from migrating
    4.   Avoid establishing large refugee camps
    5.   Establish a health information system
    6.   Ensure resources provided do not further divide communities
    7.   Focus on disease prevention

8. Work through existing structures and institutions
9. Insist that women control the distribution of relief supplies
10. Ensure open communication and coordination

B. **Implementation Principles**

1. Address identified needs in underserved areas
2. Encourage local participation
3. Integrate beneficiaries into program planning
4. Collaborate with all stakeholders
5. Coordinate with all implementing partners
6. Plan comprehensive approaches
7. Develop community-based programs
8. Make inter-sectoral linkages (sector-wide approaches)
9. Use existing resources
10. Leverage outside resources of donors and private sector
11. Build on existing platforms
12. Apply international best practices
13. Target vulnerable populations
14. Focus on high impact activities
15. Ensure equitable access to services
16. Provide assistance acceptable to beneficiaries
17. Implement with cultural sensitivity
18. Reduce the local burden of disease
19. Enhance capacities
20. Reduce vulnerabilities
21. Alleviate poverty
22. Avoid dependency
23. Foster sustainable development
24. Support governmental priorities
25. Operate cost-effectively, transparently, and accountably

C. **Implementation Mechanics**

1. Reallocation of existing local & national resources
2. Revision/refinement of present (medical) practices
    a. use of essential drugs
    b. use of standardized case management
    c. elimination of dated practices
3. Financial assistance (critical funding)
4. Technical assistance (critical skills)
    a. complement donated goods
    b. support appropriate technology
    c. develop information systems
5. Material assistance (critical goods)
    a. essential drugs and vaccines
    b. consumable supplies
    c. other stated needs of health authorities
6. Direct service provision (substitution)
7. Coordination of external assistance
    NB cooperation = shared goals; coordination = shared tasks; collaboration = shared resources
    a. identification and registration of actors
    b. actor/area/activity (who/what/where) matrix
    c. gap analysis and priority setting
    d. establishment of rapid response mechanism

      e.   gap filling via complementary inputs linking iNGOs & local NGOs to local health authorities
          (1)   technical
          (2)   material
          (3)   financial
      f.   identification of deliverables and timetables
      g.   consolidated reporting and dissemination
          (1)   group terms of reference
          (2)   meeting minutes
          (3)   epidemiology updates
          (4)   health sitreps
          (5)   component analysis
          (6)   field documentation (toolkit) for new arrivals

8.   Capacity building of host authorities
9.   Civil society partnership and support
      a.   organize community leaders
      b.   encourage gender mainstreaming
      c.   encourage privatization
      d.   discourage entitlements
10. Advocacy
11. Transition to early recovery

D.   **Strategy for Livelihood/Economic Relief**

1.   Restore productive assets (supply side interventions)
      a.   in-kind donations (e.g. food, seeds, tools, fishing nets, etc.)
      b.   types of community projects in food-for-assets programs
          (1)   natural resources development
              (a)   water harvesting
              (b)   soil conservation
          (2)   restoration of agri(aqua)culture potential
              (a)   irrigation systems
              (b)   seed systems
          (3)   infrastructure rehabilitation
              (a)   schools
              (b)   market places
              (c)   community granaries
              (d)   warehouses
              (e)   roads
              (f)   bridges
          (4)   diversification of livelihoods
              (a)   training and experience sharing

2.   Increase individual purchasing power
      a.   cash distribution
      b.   cash for work (cash for assets)
      c.   vouchers
      d.   micro-credit
      e.   job fairs
      f.   artisanal production
      g.   livelihoods/income generation

3.   Support market resumption
      a.   market rehabilitation
      b.   infrastructure rehabilitation
      c.   micro-finance institutions

E.   **Strategy for Early Recovery**

Goals—protect what's left (1 month), restore the system (6 months), improve the system (6 months)
1.   Adopt systems approach
    a.   health services
    b.   health workforce
    c.   medical logistics (drugs, vaccines, equipment, supplies, & technology)
    d.   health information system
    e.   health financing
    f.   leadership & governance
2.   Phase in assistance to beneficiaries
    a.   technical assistance
    b.   material assistance
        (1)   food
        (2)   non-food items
    c.   financial assistance
        (1)   cash grants
        (2)   cash for work
        (3)   microfinance (loans)
        (4)   livelihood/income generation
3.   Ensure responsible resource management
    a.   human resources management
        (1)   incident management command and control
        (2)   team structure and function
        (3)   staff selection
            (a)   internationals
            (b)   homologues
        (4)   field activities
            (a)   briefing
            (b)   meetings and reports
            (c)   debriefing
        (5)   operations support
            (a)   comms
            (b)   transport
            (c)   office
            (d)   food and lodging
        (6)   personal health maintenance and morale
    b.   material resources management
    c.   financial resources management
    d.   supervision
    e.   monitoring and evaluation
4.   Scale up coverage of priority health interventions
5.   Address bottlenecks of the disrupted health system (otherwise temporary solutions become permanent)
6.   Protect essential public health infrastructures
7.   Build capacity of local authorities with focus on sustainable systems
    a.   technical oversight—hiring of local experts
    b.   material assistance—production of key commodities
    c.   financial assistance
8.   Provide incentives for host government
9.   Support host country non-beneficiary population
10.   Find new partners in the development community
11.   Use health Sustainable Development Goals as targets for recovery activities
12.   Seek opportunities and develop mechanisms for transition and phase out

F. **Program Constraints and Failures**

    1. Programmatic constraints

        a. staff

            (1) western trained

            (2) hospital-based

            (3) resource intensive

            (4) technology dependent

            (5) procedurally oriented

            (6) invasive

            (7) monolingual

            (8) hazard naïve

        b. supervision

            (1) limited responsibility

            (2) limited authority

            (3) limited accountability

        c. projects

            (1) acute

            (2) curative

            (3) short-term

            (4) intermittent

        d. systems

            (1) inadequate security

            (2) weak rule of law

            (3) limited accountability framework

            (4) uncoordinated humanitarian action

    2. Project feasibility constraints

        a. security

        b. political

        c. administrative

        d. logistical

        e. technical

        f. economic

        g. developmental

    3. Hazard-specific constraints (complex emergencies)

        a. hostile armed elements

        b. limited access

        c. overburdened provincial services

        d. limited information on beneficiaries

V. **HUMANITARIAN FINANCING** [3]

A. **Shrink the Needs**

B. **Deepen the Resource Base**

C. **Improve Delivery** (Grand Bargain [4] on Efficiency)

    1. Transparency

    2. Frontline responders

    3. Cash-based programming

    4. Management cost reductions

    5. Joint and impartial needs assessments

    6. Participation revolution—including beneficiaries in decision-making

    7. Multi-year humanitarian funding

    8. Fewer earmarks

    9. Harmonized/simplified reporting

    10. Engagement between relief and development actors

VI. RESILIENCE (hazards + environment + infrastructure + institutions + livelihoods)

A. Comprehensive Disaster Risk Management

1. DRM/DRR (where risk = hazard × vulnerability; also likelihood × impact)
2. Hazard and vulnerability analysis
3. Hazard and structural mitigation (e.g. climate change adaptation plans)
4. Disaster plans
   a. all-hazard plans vs. hazard-specific plans
   b. preparedness plans
   c. contingency plans
   d. evacuation plans
   e. repurposing plans
   f. business continuity plans
   g. recovery plans
   h. R2D considerations
5. Early warning/early action systems
6. Emergency operation centers
7. Emergency relief supply systems
8. Disaster simulation exercises, tabletops, drills

B. Political

1. Proactive legislation and policy (not reactive)
2. Clear non-overlapping mandates
3. Funding commitment to comprehensive disaster management
4. Vertical and horizontal linkages in policy implementation
5. Comprehensive approaches to ecosystem protection rather than fragmentation based upon political jurisdictions
6. Generic approaches to managing technical (best) practices, but local approaches to managing community vulnerabilities
7. Communication and cooperation enabled between public and private sector, national level and local communities, and individual jurisdictions

C. Socioeconomic

1. Environmental impact of population growth
2. Environmental impact of dominant practices in land use and key livelihood sectors—agriculture, mining, manufacturing, pastoralism, etc.
3. Environmental and economic impact of hazard-specific zones, damages, and losses on biodiversity, ecosystems, and communities
4. Poverty alleviation and economic diversification programs
5. Inclusiveness thru use of gender disaggregated data
6. Indigenous knowledge and contribution to DRR
7. (Re)insurance mechanisms

D. Institutional

1. Leadership training programs
2. Transparent resource management
3. Open redundant communication channels

    4.   Streamlined work flows
    5.   Robust information management and information sharing
    6.   MEAL programs
    7.   Accountability frameworks
    8.   Inter-agency coordination
    9.   Partnership development

E.   **Environment and Infrastructure**

    1.   Hazard zoning
    2.   Hazard and structural mitigation
    3.   Remote sensing and early warning systems
    4.   Preventive maintenance

F.   **Community Capacities and Vulnerabilities**

    1.   Lifeline protection (key infrastructure assets and systems)
        NB food for assets (using food, cash, or vouchers) programs can help build physical assets listed below (see IV D 1 b)
        a.   security
        b.   communication
        c.   transportation
        d.   energy
        e.   environmental health (e.g. water supply, food security, shelter and housing)
        f.   public health (e.g. disease surveillance, primary prevention)
        g.   health
           (1)   safe hospitals program
        h.   education to achieve a literate and informed public
        i.   information and DRR technologies
    2.   Social protection and safety nets (focus on women, vulnerable groups)
    3.   Livelihood protection

VII. DEVELOPMENT PROGRAMS

A.   **Strategic Objectives** (USAID Policy Framework for Bilateral Foreign Aid [5])

    1.   Promote transformational development
        Support far-reaching, fundamental changes in relatively stable developing countries, with emphasis on improvements in governance and institutions, human capacity, and economic structure, so that countries can sustain further economic and social progress without depending on foreign aid. Focus on those countries with significant need for assistance and with adequate (or better) commitment to ruling justly, promoting economic freedom, and investing in people.
    2.   Strengthen fragile states
        Reduce fragility and establish the foundation for development progress by supporting stabilization, reform, and capacity development in fragile states when and where U.S. assistance can make a significant difference.
    3.   Support strategic states
        Help achieve major U.S. foreign policy goals in specific countries of high priority from a strategic standpoint.
    4.   Provide humanitarian relief
        Help meet immediate human needs, save lives, and alleviate suffering in countries afflicted by violent conflict, crisis, natural disasters, or persistent dire poverty.
    5.   Address global issues
        HIV/AIDS, other infectious diseases, climate change, direct support for international trade agreements, and counter narcotics.

B. **Approaches** (USAID Gender Equality and Female Empowerment Policy [6])

    1. Adopt inclusive approach
    2. Integrate gender equality into all work
    3. Build partnerships
    4. Harness science, technology, and innovation
    5. Address unique challenges in crises and conflict-affected communities
    6. Serve as thought leader
    7. Be accountable

C. **Partnership Mechanisms** (US National Strategy for Pandemic Influenza [7])

    1. International cooperation to protect lives and health
    2. Timely and sustained high-level political leadership to the disease
    3. Transparency in reporting of cases of disease in humans and in animals caused by strains that have pandemic potential to increase understanding, enhance preparedness, and ensure rapid and timely response to potential outbreaks
    4. Immediate sharing of epidemiological data and clinical samples with the World Health Organization (WHO) and the international community to characterize the nature and evolution of any outbreaks as quickly as possible
    5. Prevention and containment of an incipient epidemic through capacity building and in-country collaboration with international partners
    6. Rapid response to the first signs of accelerated disease transmission
    7. Work in a manner supportive of key multilateral organizations (WHO, FAO, OIE)
    8. Timely coordination of bilateral and multilateral resource allocations; dedication of domestic resources (human and financial); improvements in public awareness; and development of economic and trade contingency plans
    9. Increased coordination and harmonization of preparedness, prevention, response and containment activities among nations
   10. Actions based on the best available science

D. **Program Innovations at Community Level**

    1. Community interventions
       a. sector-wide approaches (SWAps)
       b. integrated health interventions
          (1) PHC
          (2) SPHC
          (3) IMCI
       c. home-based interventions
          (1) CTC
       d. microfinance
          (1) Grameen Bank
    2. Best practice program models (centers of excellence arising within a community)
       a. Matlab Health Research Center (part of ICDDR, Bangladesh)
       b. Shoklo Malaria Research Unit, Tak Province, Thailand
       c. Fistula Hospital, Addis Ababa, Ethiopia
       d. Behrhorst Clinic, Guatemala
    3. Self-replicating centers of excellence
       a. Fistula Hospital, Addis Ababa, Ethiopia

VIII.   SEEDS OF CHANGE

    A.   **Innovators**

    B.   **Thought Leaders**

    C.   **Change Agents**

    D.   **Early Adopters**

    E.   **Craft Groups**

    F.   **Centers of Excellence**

    G.   **Communities of Practice**

    H.   **Global Alliance**

    I.   **Crowds**

References

1. Inter-agency Standing Committee. *Guidance Note on Using the Cluster Approach to Strengthen Humanitarian Response*. Retrieved November 24, 2006 from https://interagencystandingcommittee.org/system/files/legacy_files/Cluster%20implementation%2C%20Guidance%20Note%2C%20WG66%2C%2020061115-.pdf.
2. OCHA. Global Cluster Leads (as of June 2012). Available from http://reliefweb.int/sites/reliefweb.int/files/resources/map_2809.pdf.
3. High-Level Panel on Humanitarian Financing Report to the United Nations Secretary-General. *Too important to fail—Addressing the humanitarian financing gap*. Available from https://interagencystandingcommittee.org/grand-bargain-hosted-iasc/documents/too-important-fail-addressing-humanitarian-financing-gap-high.
4. Australian Aid, Belgian Development Corporation, Government of Bulgaria, Government of Canada, et al. *The Grand Bargain—a shared commitment to better serve people in need*. Available from https://interagencystandingcommittee.org/system/files/grand_bargain_final_22_may_final-2.pdf.
5. USAID. Policy framework for bilateral foreign aid. January 2006. Available from USAID's Development Experience Clearinghouse https://www.dec.usaid.gov, and https://www.usaid.gov/sites/default/files/documents/1868/201mam.pdf.
6. USAID. Gender equality and female empowerment policy. Available from https://www.usaid.gov/sites/default/files/documents/1865/GenderEqualityPolicy_0.pdf.
7. US Homeland Security Council. National strategy for pandemic influenza. Available from http://www.flu.gov/planning-preparedness/federal/pandemic-influenza.pdf.

Annex 8.2
SECURITY SECTOR

I. DEFINITIONS (Rome Statute [1])

A. **Crimes** (within the International Criminal Court's Jurisdiction) (Article 5)

1. Genocide (Article 6)—acts committed with intent to destroy, in whole or in part, a national, ethnic, racial, or religious group
   a. killing members of the group
   b. causing serious bodily or mental harm to members of the group
   c. inflicting on the group conditions of life calculated to bring about its physical destruction in whole or in part
   d. imposing measures intended to prevent births within the group
   e. forcibly transferring children of the group to another group
2. Crimes against humanity (Article 7)—acts committed as part of a widespread or systematic attack against any civilian population, with knowledge of the attack
   a. murder
   b. extermination
   c. enslavement
   d. deportation
   e. imprisonment in violation of international law
   f. torture
   g. rape, sexual slavery, enforced prostitution, forced pregnancy, enforced sterilization, or other comparable form of sexual violence
   h. persecution on political, racial, national, ethnic, cultural, religious, gender, or other grounds universally recognized as impermissible under international law
   i. enforced disappearance
   j. apartheid
   k. other inhumane acts intentionally causing great suffering or serious injury to body or to mental or physical health
3. War crimes (Article 8)
   a. grave breaches of the Geneva Conventions of 12 Aug 1949
      (1) willful killing
      (2) torture or inhumane treatment including biological experiments
      (3) willfully causing great suffering
      (4) extensive destruction and appropriation of property
      (5) compelling a POW to serve in the armed forces of a hostile power
      (6) willfully depriving a POW of the right to a fair trial
      (7) unlawful deportation
      (8) taking of hostages
   b. serious violations of laws and customs applicable in international armed conflict
      (1) intentionally directing attacks against the civilian population or against civilians not taking direct part in hostilities
      (2) intentionally directing attacks against civilian objects
      (3) intentionally directing attacks against personnel, installations, material, units, or vehicles involved in humanitarian assistance or peacekeeping mission
      (4) intentionally launching an attack in the knowledge that it will cause incidental civilian loss of life or severe damage to the natural environment
      (5) attacking undefended towns, villages, dwellings, or buildings which are not military targets
      (6) killing or wounding a combatant who has surrendered
      (7) improper use of a flag of truce, flag or insignia or uniform of the enemy or of the UN, or emblems of the Geneva conventions resulting in death or serious personal injury

      (8)   transfer by the Occupying Power of parts of its own civilian population into the territory it occupies, or the deportation or transfer of all or parts of the population of the occupied territory within or outside the territory

      (9)   intentionally directing attacks against buildings dedicated to religion, education, art, science, charitable purposes, historic monuments, hospitals, and places where sick are collected, provided they are not military objectives

   (10)   subjecting persons to physical mutilation or to medical or scientific experiments which are not justified by the medical treatment nor carried out in his/her interest

   (11)   killing or wounding treacherously individuals belonging to the hostile nation or army

   (12)   declaring that no quarter will be given

   (13)   destroying or seizing the enemy's property unless such be imperatively demanded by the necessities of war

   (14)   declaring abolished, suspended, or inadmissible in a court of law the rights and actions of the nationals of the hostile party

   (15)   compelling the nationals of the hostile party to take part in the operations of war directed against their own country

   (16)   pillaging a town or place, even when taken by assault

   (17)   employing poison or poison weapons

   (18)   employing asphyxiating, poisonous or other gases, and all analogous liquids, materials, or devices

   (19)   employing bullets which expand or flatten easily in the human body

   (20)   employing weapons, projectiles, material and methods of warfare which cause superfluous injury or unnecessary suffering

   (21)   committing outrages upon personal dignity, in particular humiliating and degrading treatment

   (22)   committing rape, sexual slavery, enforced prostitution, forced pregnancy, enforced sterilization, or other comparable form of sexual violence

   (23)   utilizing a civilian or other protected person to render certain areas or military forces immune from military operations

   (24)   intentionally directing attacks against buildings, material, medical units, transport, and personnel using the emblems of the Geneva Conventions in conformity with international law

   (25)   conscripting or enlisting children under the age of 15 years

  c.   serious violations of common article 3 applicable in non-international armed conflict, i.e. acts vs. persons taking no active part in the hostilities, including armed forces placed hors de combat by sickness, wounds, detention, or other cause

    (1)   violence to life and person

    (2)   outrages upon personal dignity

    (3)   taking of hostages

    (4)   passing of sentences and carrying out of executions

  d.   non-applicability of c (above) to internal disturbances (riots, sporadic violence, etc.)

  e.   other serious violations of laws and customs applicable in non-international armed conflict

4.   Crime of aggression (provision to be adopted)

II.   SECURITY OBJECTIVES

A.   Unimpeded Access to Beneficiaries

1.   Registration/verification
2.   Protection
3.   Humanitarian assistance
4.   Family reunification
5.   Information dissemination

B. **Security for Refugees and Humanitarian Personnel**

C. **Law Enforcement** (perpetrators of violence are arrested, charged, and tried in a civil court of law)

D. **Free and Informed Choices**

E. **Program Participation of Beneficiaries** (especially women)

F. **Relocation** (only if voluntary, people are medically fit, and families are united)

III. DISCRIMINATION PRETEXTS

A. **Age**

B. **Gender**

C. **Race**

D. **Religion**

E. **Ethnicity**

F. **Geographic Origin**

G. **Socioeconomic Status**

H. **Sexual Orientation**

I. **Disability Status**

J. **HIV Status**

K. **Migratory Status**

L. **Forced Displacement**

IV. ROLE OF HIC/OSOCC/CMOC

A. **Access Negotiations**

B. **GIS, Maps, and Analysis**

C. **Interagency Convoys**

D. **Pipeline Monitoring**

E. **Contingency Planning**

V. HEALTH CONSEQUENCES OF SECURITY BREAKDOWN

A. **Decreased Access and Protection for Beneficiaries**

B. **Increased Morbidity and Mortality**

    1. Direct trauma
    2. Diseases of overcrowding and displacement
    3. Outbreaks of preventable and controlled diseases
    4. Untreated chronic illnesses
    5. Excess mortality in affected population

C.   **Degradation of Health System**

1.   Degradation/destruction of health infrastructure
2.   Degradation/disruption of health services
3.   Attrition of health personnel
4.   Disruption of medical logistics
5.   Increased demand for health financing
6.   Weaknesses in health governance

D.   **Loss of Human Capital and Physical Assets**

E.   **Loss of Development Opportunity**

Reference

1. Rome Statute of the International Criminal Court, July 17, 1998, 2187 U.N.T.S. 90. Available from: http://untreaty.un.org/cod/icc/statute/romefra.htm.

Annex 8.3
HEALTH SECTOR

Glossary

ABX	antibiotics
AFP	acute flaccid paralysis
AIDS	acquired immune deficiency syndrome
ASDR	age-specific death rate
BCG	bacillus Calmette-Guérin
BMI	body mass index
c	with
cc	cubic centimeter
CDR	crude death rate
CFR	case fatality ratio
CI	confidence interval
cm	centimeter
CSS	cluster sample survey
CTC	community therapeutic care (malnutrition management program)
d	day
D5	dextrose 5% in water
D10	dextrose 10% in water
D&C	dilation and curettage
D_{eff}	design effect
DTP	diphtheria + tetanus + pertussis vaccine
DRR	disaster risk reduction
EOC	Emergency Operations Center
EPI	Expanded Programme on Immunization
gm	gram
GAM	global acute malnutrition
gtt	drops
h	hour
H	height
HAM	height-for-age median
HAZ	height-for-age z score
HB	hepatitis B
HCW	health care worker
HH	household
Hib	*Haemophilus influenzae* type b
HIV	human immunodeficiency virus
ICDDR	International Centre for Diarrhoeal Disease Research, Bangladesh
ICS	incident command system
ID	infectious disease
IMCI	Integrated Management of Childhood Illness (WHO initiative)
IMPAC	Integrated Management of Pregnancy and Childbirth (WHO initiative)
IMR	infant mortality rate
IPD	inpatient department
IV	intravenous
kg	kilogram
L	liter
L&D	labor and delivery
m	meter
MAM	moderate acute malnutrition
MCI	mass casualty incident

MCV	measles-containing vaccine
MD	medical doctor
mg	milligram
MISP	Minimum Initial Service Package (used in reproductive health)
mL	milliliter
MMR	measles + mumps + rubella vaccine
mo	month
MR	measles + rubella vaccine
MSF	Médecins sans Frontières
MUAC	mid-upper arm circumference
NGO	non-governmental organization
NGT	nasogastric tube
NID	national immunization day(s)
NL	normal
NS	normal saline
O10	over 10 year-old
OPD	outpatient department
OPV	oral polio vaccine
OR	operating room
ORS	oral rehydration solution
OTP	outpatient therapeutic program
PCV	pneumococcal conjugate vaccine
PO	by mouth
ppm	parts per million
RL	Ringer's lactate
RUSF	ready-to-use supplementary food
RUTF	ready-to-use therapeutic food
RV	rotavirus
Rx	medication
SAM	severe acute malnutrition
SC	stabilization center
SD	standard deviation
SFC	supplementary feeding center
SFP	supplementary feeding program
SIA	supplemental immunization activities
SOP	standard operating procedure
t	teaspoon
T	tablespoon
TB	tuberculosis
TFC	therapeutic feeding center
Tx	treatment
U5	under 5 year-old
U5DR	under 5 year-old death rate
U5MR	under 5 year-old mortality rate
U10	under 10 year-old
W	weight
W/H	weight-for-height
WHM	weight-for-height median
WHO	World Health Organization
WHZ	weight-for-height z score
wk	week
YF	yellow fever
yr	year

I.   DISASTER HEALTH CORE DISCIPLINES

A.   Clinical Medicine

1. Prehospital care
2. Primary, preventive, and basic services
   a. comprehensive primary health care
   b. child health services
   c. reproductive health services
   d. trauma services
   e. mental health services
   f. chronic diseases
   g. infection control
3. Referral care

B.   Public Health

1. Rapid epidemiological assessment (minimum essential data sets)
2. Inter-agency health coordination
3. Standardized case management
4. Environmental health (minimum standards)
5. Epidemic preparedness and response
6. Disease surveillance (surveillance case definitions, data flow, and analysis)
7. Special surveys (cluster sample surveys)
8. Health policy and personnel planning
9. Immunization programs (EPI)
10. Medical logistics

C.   Disaster Management

1. Site security
2. Urban search and rescue
3. Hazard-specific issues (hazard analysis, mitigation, vulnerability reduction)
4. Disaster response modalities (ICS/EOC)
5. Geographic information systems
6. Public information
7. Community recovery

D.   WHO Mandated Responsibilities in Disaster

1. Core functions (World Health Assembly Res 58.1)
   a. needs assessment
   b. health coordination
   c. gap filling
   d. capacity building
   NB protection & nutrition are beyond the mandate of WHO
2. Critical functions in emergency response (WHO *Emergency Response Framework*)
   a. leadership
   b. information
   c. technical expertise
   d. core services

II.   PRIMARY HEALTH CARE PROGRAMS

A.   Primary Health Care (Alma Ata Declaration [1])

1. Health Education
2. Food and Nutrition

      3.   Water and Sanitation
      4.   Maternal and Child Health, Family Planning
      5.   Immunization
      6.   Prevention of Endemic Disease
      7.   Treatment of Common Disease and Injury
      8.   Essential Drugs

  B.   **Selective Primary Health Care** (Walsh and Warren [2])

      1.   Growth Monitoring
      2.   Oral Rehydration Therapy
      3.   Breast Feeding
      4.   Immunization
      5.   Female Literacy
      6.   Family Planning
      7.   Food Supplements

III. DISEASE PREVENTION

  A.   **Definitions**

      1.   Primary (individual without disease)
          Goal—prevent the disease from starting (consider host-agent-environment)
          a.   limit pathogenesis of a disease-causing agent (e.g. lower cholesterol levels)
          b.   alter the environment to keep the disease from humans (e.g. regulate asbestos exposures)
          c.   strengthen host resistance to the disease (e.g. measles immunization, water fluoridation)
      2.   Secondary (individual with disease but without symptoms)
          Goal—prevent disease symptoms and complications from developing
          a.   intervene after exposure (e.g. rabies vaccination)
          b.   detect and treat disease before it becomes symptomatic (e.g. cancer screening)
          c.   prevent disease spread by treating contacts (e.g. TB exposure treatment)
      3.   Tertiary (individual with symptomatic disease)
          Goal—cure or control of clinical disease (bulk of clinical medicine)
          a.   cure disease or reverse clinical manifestations (e.g. appendectomy, thrombolysis)
          b.   control disease progression to avoid complications (e.g. retroviral drugs, anticoagulation in atrial fibrillation)
          c.   control spread of disease to others (e.g. TB case management)

  B.   **Great Public Health Achievements—US, 1900–9999** (CDC [3])

      1.   Vaccination
      2.   Motor-vehicle safety
      3.   Safer workplaces
      4.   Control of infectious diseases
      5.   Decline in deaths from coronary heart disease and stroke
      6.   Safer and healthier foods
      7.   Healthier mothers and babies
      8.   Family planning
      9.   Fluoridation of drinking water
     10. Recognition of tobacco use as a health hazard

  C.   **Great Public Health Achievements—US, 2001–2010** (CDC [4])

      1.   Vaccine-preventable diseases
      2.   Prevention and control of infectious diseases
      3.   Tobacco control

4. Maternal and infant health
5. Motor vehicle safety
6. Cardiovascular disease prevention
7. Occupational safety
8. Cancer prevention
9. Childhood lead poisoning prevention
10. Public health preparedness and response

D. **Vaccinations**

1. Infant schedule (WHO)

Table 8.3.1
Infant Vaccination Schedule

Age	Vaccine
Birth	BCG, HB-1, $\pm$ OPV birth dose
6 wks	DTP-1, OPV/IPV-1, HB-2, Hib-1, PCV-1, RV-1
10 wks	DTP-2, OPV/IPV-2, HB-3, Hib-2, PCV-2, RV-2
14 wks	DTP-3, OPV/IPV-3, HB-4, Hib-3, PCV-3, RV-3
9–12 mo	MCV-1 (e.g. MR or MMR)
15 mo	MCV-2

NB   Table does not convey all options for vaccine administration.
Diphtheria toxoid is not manufactured as monovalent vaccine. It is combined with tetanus tox-oid—either full-strength dose for pediatric use (DT), or reduced-strength dose for adult use (Td). These are combined with acellular or whole-cell pertussis antigens—either full-strength dose for pediatric use (DTaP, DTwP), or reduced-strength dose for adolescent/adult use (Tdap).
DTP-1 is a good indicator of access to care.
DTP-3 is a good indicator of ultimate service delivery.

2. Immunization program

Table 8.3.2
Immunization Program Components

Intervention	Polio	Measles
Routine immunization	+	+
Supplementary immunization	National immunization days (NID)	Supplementary immunization activities (SIA)
Surveillance	Acute flaccid paralysis (AFP)	Case-based
Case follow-up	Mop-up campaign	Case management

3. Vaccine quantities

Table 8.3.3
Calculation of Vaccine Quantities

Indicator & benchmark	Quantity
Total population	100,000
Target population (6 mo–15 yr) 45% total	45,000
Cover objective = 100%	45,000
Number of doses (1 for measles)	45,000
Expected loss 15%	52,940
Increase reserve by 25%	66,175
Round up	67,000

IV. CLINICAL FACILITIES

A. Generic Profile

		Fixed Clinics	Health Centers	Dist Hospitals
1.	Quantity			
2.	Catchment population	5–10k	<50k	100k
3.	Access to facility	self	self	by referral
4.	Staffing			
	a. quantity (~1/1000 p)	2–5 staff	5–10 staff	variable
	b. skill mix	1 HCW	5 HCW, 1 MD	5 MD, 1 surg
5.	Caseload (% of catchment population/d)	1–10%	1–10%	
6.	Bed capacity (10/10,000 population)			
7.	Bed occupancy			
8.	Referral load (% of caseload)	10%	10%	
9.	Referral system			
10.	Clinical services	OPD, ORS	→ + IPD, L&D	→ + OR

a. departments/units (verify functioning of expected services)

		Fixed Clinics	Health Centers	Dist Hospitals
(1)	clinical			
	(a) OPD	+	+	+
	(b) IPD	–	+	+
	(c) L&D	–	+	+
	(d) surgery	–	+/–	+
	(e) other			
(2)	dispensary	+/–	+	+
(3)	diagnostic lab	+/–	+	+
(4)	blood bank	–	–	+
(5)	radiology	–	–	+

V. REPRODUCTIVE HEALTH

A. Safe Motherhood (IMPAC, MISP)

NB 15% of pregnant women have complications requiring emergency OB care; 5% (3–7%) need C-section; 10% of deliveries will have primary post-partum hemorrhage within 24 h

1. Causes of maternal death — Time to death
   a. other emergencies 22%   ruptured uterus—1 d
   b. hemorrhage 18%   ante-partum—12 h, post-partum—2 h
   c. eclampsia 12%   2 d
   d. obstructed labor 8%   3 d
   e. sepsis 9%   6 d
   f. unsafe abortion 18%   variable
   g. other indirect (malaria, HIV) 13% variable
2. Basic emergency obstetric care (1 facility/125k pop)
   a. parenteral antibiotics
   b. parenteral oxytocics
   c. parenteral anticonvulsants for pre-eclampsia & eclampsia
   d. manual removal of placenta
   e. removal of retained products (vacuum aspiration, D&C)
   f. assisted vaginal delivery (vacuum, forceps)
3. Comprehensive emergency obstetric care (as above plus below) (1 facility/500k pop)
   a. Caesarean section (5–15% of deliveries)
   b. blood transfusion

4. Treatment of obstructed labor
    a. McRoberts maneuver—flex thighs at the hips and push knees to maternal abdomen
    b. pressure on suprapubic area
    c. proctoepisiotomy
    d. Wood's corkscrew maneuver—rotate shoulders 180° or to an oblique diameter to disengage the impacted shoulder
    e. delivery of the posterior arm (>incidence of humerus and clavicle fractures)
    f. symphysiotomy
    g. Zavanelli maneuver—replace head into the vagina and perform C-section
5. Essential newborn care
    a. basic newborn resuscitation
    b. warmth (drying and kangaroo care)
    c. eye prophylaxis (tetracycline ointment)
    d. clean cord care
    e. early and exclusive breast feeding

VI. WATER AND SANITATION

A. **Classification** (D Mara, R Feachem [5])

Table 8.3.4
Environmental Classification of Water & Excreta-Related Diseases

Diseases	Pathogen/disease	Preventive Measures
Fecal-oral = water-borne + water-washed	virus—hepatitis A/E/F, polio, rotavirus, adenovirus	water-washed: > H_2O quantity water-borne: > H_2O quality
	bacteria—*Campylobacter, E. coli, Salmonella, Shigella, Vibrio*	
	protozoa—*Entamoeba, Balantidium, Cryptosporidium, Giardia, Isospora*	
	helminths—*Ascaris, Enterobius*	
Non-fecal-oral water-washed	skin infections—scabies, leprosy, yaws	> H_2O quantity; > hygiene education
	eye infections—trachoma, conjunctivitis	
	louse-borne fevers	
Water-based	bacteria—*Leptospira, Francisella, Legionella*	< contact with contaminated H_2O
	helminths—*Schistosoma, Clonorchis, Fasciola, Paragonimus, Dracunculus*	
Insect-vectored, water-related mosquitoes (breeding in water), flies (biting/breeding near water)	malaria, dengue, Rift Valley fever, Japanese encephalitis, yellow fever, sleeping sickness, oncho, filariasis	destroy breeding sites; use barrier precautions (ITNs)
Insect-vectored, excreta-related flies, cockroaches	includes all fecal-oral diseases + water-based helminths + geohelminths + taeniasis	
Rodent-vectored	similar to insect-vectored, excreta-related but includes all water-based pathogens listed (except *Legionella*)	> rodent control; < contact with contaminated H_2O
Geohelminths	roundworm, hookworm, whipworm	excreta disposal
Taenia	beef and pork tapeworm	excreta disposal; proper meat cooking

Source: D Mara, R Feachem in *Journal of Environmental Engineering* © 1999. Used with permission of ASCE

B.   **Prevention** (adapted from R Feachem [6])

Table 8.3.5
Water & Excreta-related Disease Prevention Measures

Disease	Prevention Measures						
	H$_2$O quality	H$_2$O quantity	Excreta disposal	Excreta Tx	Personal hygiene	Waste H$_2$O disposal	Food hygiene
Diarrheal disease & enteric fevers							
Viral	2	2	1	1	2	0	1
Bacterial	3	3	2	1	3	0	3
Protozoal	1	3	2	1	3	0	2
Polio, Hepatitis A	1	3	2	1	3	0	1
Water-washed (skin, eye, louse-borne disease)	0	3	0	0	3	0	0
Water-based							
Schisto	1	1	3	2	1	0	0
Guinea worm	3	0	0	0	0	0	0
Clonorchis	0	0	2	2	0	0	3
Water-related							
Malaria	0	0	0	0	0	1	0
Dengue, YF	0	0	0	0	0	1	0
Filariasis	0	0	3	0	0	3	0
Worms without intermediate host	0	1	3	2	1	0-1	1–2
Worms with intermediate host	0	0	3	3	0	0	3

Source: R Feachem in *Water Supply and Sanitation in Developing Countries* © 1983. Used with permission of Chartered Institution of Water and Environmental Management
0 = no importance; 3 = great importance

A range of generic prevention measures should be considered for its impact on diseases in a biological "all-hazards" environment. Overall, excreta disposal, water quantity, personal hygiene, and food hygiene commonly contribute more to environmental health than do other listed measures. Epidemic threats will oblige heightened consideration of disease-specific strategies for prevention and control.

C.   **Water Treatment (bold of particular relevance in clinical facilities)**

1 ppm = 1 mg/kg (solids)

= 1 mg/L (liquids) = 1 μg/mL (liquids) = basic unit of measure for chloroscopes

∴   10,000 ppm = 1%

Table 8.3.6
Chlorine Concentration and Uses

PPM	Equivalents	Concentration %	Use
0.5	0.5 mg/L 0.0005 g/L, mg/mL 0.00005 g/100 mL	0.00005%	piped water systems, goal for all end user drinking water
1	1 mg/L 0.001 g/L, mg/mL 0.0001 g/100 mL	0.0001%	standpost systems
2	2 mg/L 0.002 g/L, mg/mL 0.0002 g/100 mL	0.0002%	pre-treatment for selected/known water sources—tanker trucks at filling stations, protected tube wells, clear rainwater
5	5 mg/L .0.005 g/L, mg/mL 0.0005 g/100 mL	0.0005%	pre-treatment for untested/unknown water sources—unprotected wells, cloudy surface water; filter/flocculate before chlorinating

PPM	Equivalents	Concentration %	Use
10	10 mg/L 0.01 g/L, mg/mL 0.001 g/100 mL	0.001%	water with known fecal contamination; filter/flocculate before chlorinating
30	30 mg/L .03 g/L, mg/mL .003 g/100 mL	0.003%	water from contaminated well or borehole (needs super-chlorination to achieve breakpoint chlorination)
50	50 mg/L 0.05 g/L, mg/mL 0.005 g/100 mL	0.005%	utensil rinse in restaurants (USA)
500	**500 mg/L** **0.5 g/L, mg/mL** **0.05 g/100 mL**	**0.05%**	**hands, skin (e.g. wash points)**
2000	**2000 mg/L** **2 g/L, mg/mL** **0.2 g/100 mL**	**0.2%** **(0.5% at ICDDR)**	**cholera cots, covers, floors, walls, equipment, clothing, isolation areas (cholera, dysentery, influenza epidemics)**
10,000	10,000 mg/L 10 g/L, mg/mL 1 g/100 mL	1%	latrine door handles
20,000	**20,000 mg/L** **20 g/L, mg/mL** **2 g/100 mL**	**2%**	**body fluids (stool, vomitus)—stool buckets, corpses (disinfection for burial), shoes (perimeter control)**
50,000	50,000 mg/L 50 g/L, mg/mL 5 g/100 mL	5%	household bleach

Table 8.3.7
Chlorine Products and Dilution

Product	Potable Water Treatment 0.0005%	Hands and Skin Cleaning 0.05%	Bedding/clothes Cleaning 0.5%	Body Fluid/corpse Cleaning 2.0%
Household bleach Sodium hypochlorite solution 5% active chlorine (50 mg/mL)	2.5 mL (0.5 t)/5 gal ≈ 8 gtt/gal, 2 gtt/L 2.5 mL × 50 mg/mL = 125 mg Cl in 20 L ≈ 6 mg/L or 6 PPM NB double if source is contaminated	100 mL in 10 L water	1 L in 10 L water	4 L in 6 L water
Bleaching powder Chlorinated lime 30% active chlorine		16 g (1 T) to 10 L water	16 g (1 T) to 1 L water	64 g (4 T) to 1 L water
High-test hypochlorite (HTH) Calcium hypochlorite Chlorine granules 70% active chlorine		7 g (0.5 T) to 10 L water	7 g (0.5 T) to 1 L water	28 g (2 T) to 1 L water

VII. FOOD AND NUTRITION

Malnutrition is #1 risk to child health worldwide. It contributes to an estimated 2.5 M out of 6.3 M U5 deaths/year.

A.   **Prediction and Early Warning Systems**

1.   FEWS NET products
  a.   Food Security Outlook (FSO)—assumptions and 8-mo projections issued 3×/year
  b.   Food Security Outlook Update (FSOU)—update mid-term between FSOs
  c.   Key Messages (KM)—precedes FSO
  d.   Price Bulletin (PB)
  e.   Food Assistance Outlook Brief (FAOB)—regional outlook

2. FEWS NET distribution calendar
   a. January—Key Messages (KM)
   b. **February—Food Security Outlook (FSO)**
   c. March—Key Messages (KM)
   d. April—Food Security Outlook Update (FSOU)
   e. May—Key Messages (KM)
   f. **June—Food Security Outlook (FSO)**
   g. July—Key Messages (KM)
   h. August—Food Security Outlook Update (FSOU)
   i. September—Key Messages (KM)
   j. **October—Food Security Outlook (FSO)**
   k. November—Key Messages (KM)
   l. December—Food Security Outlook Update (FSOU) (optional)

B. **Protein-calorie Malnutrition**

   1. Screening
      U5—mid-upper arm circumference (MUAC) used as a screening tool in pedes and adults. In pedes, < 13.5 cm or edema is referred for W/H measurements.
   2. Individual diagnosis
      a. pedes (U10)
         anthropometrics: ΔW/H before ΔW/Age before ΔH/Age
         Acute   <–>   Chronic

Table 8.3.8
Anthropometric Indicators in Children

Combined Anthropometrics		W/H % of Median	
		>80% (NL)	<80%
H/Age % of Median	>90% (NL)	NL	Wasted
	<90%	Stunted	Wasted & stunted
Acute Malnutrition (Wasting)	**W/H Z Score** (WHZ)	**W/H % of Median** (WHM)	**MUAC** (cm) (6–59 mo)
Mild acute	$-2 \leq z < -1$	80% $\leq$ % WHM < 90%	12.5 $\leq$ MUAC < 13.5
Moderate acute (MAM)	$-3 \leq z < -2$	70% $\leq$ % WHM < 80%	11.5 $\leq$ MUAC < 12.5
Severe acute (SAM)	$z < -3$ or symmetrical edema	WHM < 70% or symmetrical edema	MUAC < 11.5 or symmetrical edema
Global acute (GAM)	$z < -2$ or symmetrical edema	WHM < 80% or symmetrical edema	MUAC < 12.5 or symmetrical edema
Underweight	**W/Age Z Score** (WAZ)	**W/Age % of Median** (WAM)	
Mild	$-2 \leq z < -1$		
Moderate	$-3 \leq z < -2$		
Severe	$z < -3$ or symmetrical edema		
Chronic Malnutrition (Stunting)	**H/Age Z Score** (HAZ)	**H/Age % of Median** (HAM)	
Mild stunting	$-2 \leq z < -1$		
Moderately stunted	$-3 \leq z < -2$	85% $\leq$ HAM < 90%	
Severely stunted	$z < -3$ or symmetrical edema	HAM < 85% or symmetrical edema	

Note: in U2, length is the preferred term over height

Wasting

- WHO defines three types of severe malnutrition: severe wasting (SAM), severe stunting, and edematous malnutrition. This last includes kwashiorkor and marasmatic kwashiorkor in the Wellcome classification.
- SAM = severe wasting cases or bilateral pitting edema cases (where due to malnutrition)
- SAM = WHZ < −3, MUAC < 11.5 cm, or bilateral pitting edema (WHO). WHM not in definition.
- SAM prevalence worldwide ≈ 20,000,000.
- SAM mortality ≈ 9× mortality of normally nourished child and its CFR can be 10–50%.
- GAM = MAM + SAM
- GAM = moderate wasting cases, severe wasting cases, or bilateral pitting edema cases (where due to malnutrition)

Underweight

- Underweight is not used for screening or surveys in nutritional emergencies. It reflects past (chronic) and present (acute) undernutrition and is unable to distinguish between them. It encompasses children who are wasted and/or stunted. However, weight gain over time can be a sensitive indicator of growth faltering which is easily tracked on Road to Health charts.

Stunting

- Stunting generally occurs before age 2. It is irreversible.
- Stunting prevalence worldwide ≈ 165,000,000.
- Stunting is not a good predictor of mortality, but the CFR from IDs in cases of severe stunting ≈ 3× the CFR from IDs in cases without stunting.

Reference standards can be absolute MUAC, centile, % of median reference, or z scores:

- MUAC
- Easy to understand. An excellent predictor of mortality. Permits comparisons between age groups insofar as the low growth velocity of MUAC in the U5 age group makes data roughly comparable. May be used alone in "quick-and-dirty" convenience samples to estimate local prevalence of wasting. However, not used alone in authoritative anthropometric surveys, and is commonly part of a two stage screening process to determine eligibility for feeding programs.
- Centiles
  Easy to understand. Permits comparisons between age groups and outliers.
  However, data are not convenient to convert.
  E.g. z -4.0 = 0.0032nd percentile
- % of Median of reference population WHM is the preferred indicator to determine eligibility for feeding programs (Sphere). Calculations are easy and are used in the WHO Road to Health Charts.
  However, median reference data are not comparable between ages.
  eg   60% wt-for-age = severe malnutrition in infants
                             = moderate malnutrition in school age kids
  Moreover, median reference data are not comparable between indicators.
  eg   60% wt-for-age = severe malnutrition in infants
             60% wt-for-ht = death
- Z scores
  Preferred indicator (Sphere, WHO) for reporting anthropometry survey results because it permits comparisons between age groups and nutritional indices.
  However, data may be difficult to understand.
  eg   z score wt-for-age for 1 y/o:

$$= \frac{wt_{Pt} - wt_{ref\,pop}}{SD_{ref\,pop}}$$

$$= \frac{6.1kg - 10.1kg}{1.0}$$

$$= -4 \text{ SD below median for his age}$$

Overall:

WHZ gives higher prevalence of malnutrition than WHM for the same population. This is most marked where there is low baseline prevalence of disease, and especially for adolescents (who get subsequently over-referred).

WHZ is more statistically valid, but WHM is better predictor of mortality and is used for admission to TFCs.

Weight-for-age is influenced by weight-for-height and height-for-age. It can be difficult to interpret.

b. adults and adolescents (O10)

anthropometrics: BMI = weight (kg)/height (m)^2

Table 8.3.9
Anthropometric Indicators in Adults

Nutritional Status	BMI (adults & adolescents)	MUAC (cm) (adults)	MUAC (cm) (pregnant & lactating)
Obese	30+		
Overweight	25 ≤ BMI < 30		
NL	18.5 ≤ BMI < 25		
Mild malnutrition	17 ≤ BMI < 18.5		
Moderate malnutrition	16 ≤ BMI < 17	16.0 ≤ MUAC < 18.5	17.0 ≤ MUAC < 18.5
Severe malnutrition	BMI < 16 or edema or < 5% of 10–18 yr reference population	MUAC < 16.0 or edema	MUAC < 17.0 or edema
Global (mod + severe)	BMI < 17 or edema	MUAC < 18.5 or edema	MUAC < 18.5 or edema

3. Population prevalence (U5)

    a. survey key attributes

        (1) representative at unit of analysis

        (2) robust (>25 clusters recommended)

        (3) standardized (standardization test done)

        (4) data normally distributed (check standard deviation)

        (5) findings plausible (plausibility score)

    b. preferences for indicator and methods (IPC)

        (1) GAM by WHZ from representative survey >

        (2) GAM by WHZ from sentinel sites >

        (3) GAM by MUAC from representative survey >

        (4) GAM by MUAC from exhaustive screening >

        (5) GAM by MUAC from sentinel sites >

        (6) GAM by MUAC from screening

Malnutrition Classification

Table 8.3.10
Malnutrition Classification by Prevalence Range (WHO [7])

Malnutrition	Prevalence (%)			
	Acceptable (Low)	Poor (Med)	Serious (High)	Critical (Very high)
Wasting (GAM)	<5	5–9	10–14	≥15
Underweight	<10	10–19	20–29	≥30
Stunting	<20	20–29	30–39	≥40

Source: World Health Organization. In: *Global Database on Child Growth and Malnutrition* © 2017. Used with permission of WHO

Table 8.3.11
Malnutrition Classification by Prevalence Range (IPC [8])

Indicator	Prevalence (%)				
	Phase 1 Acceptable	Phase 2 Alert	Phase 3 Serious	Phase 4 Critical	Phase 5 Ext Critical
GAM by WHZ % < -2 or edema	<5	5–9.9	10–14.9	15–29.9	≥30
GAM by MUAC % < 12.5 cm or edema	<6	6–10.9		11–16.9	≥17

Source: IPC Global Partners © 2016. Used with permission of IPC Global Partnership

Acute Food Security Classification

Table 8.3.12
Area Food Security Reference Table (adapted from IPC [9])

Phase Classification	Reference Data (not all indicators required to determine classification)
Phase 1—Minimal generally food secure (green)	CDR < 0.5/10,0000/d, U5DR ≤ 1/10,000/d GAM < 5% Food consumption usually adequate (> 2100 kcal/p/d) Livelihood assets sustainable utilization
Phase 2—Stressed borderline food insecure (yellow)	CDR < 0.5/10,000/d, U5DR ≤ 1/10,000/d GAM 5–10 % Food consumption borderline adequate (2100 kcal/p/d) 20%+ of HH c livelihood assets stressed & unsustainable utilization (livelihood deficit) Non-food expenditures (schools, health care) decrease
Phase 3—Crisis acute food and livelihood crisis (orange)	CDR 0.5–1/10,000/d, U5DR 1–2/10,000/d GAM 10–15% or greater than usual and increasing 20%+ of HH c food consumption gaps (<2100 kcal/p/d or 2100 kcal/p/d via asset stripping) (survival deficit) Livelihood assets accelerated & critical depletion
Phase 4—Emergency (red)	CDR 1–2/10,000/d, U5DR > 2–4/10,000/d (excess mortality) GAM > 15–30% or greater than usual and increasing 20%+ of HH c food consumption gaps marked (< 2100 kcal/p/d) Livelihood assets near complete & irreversible depletion
Phase 5—Famine (maroon)	CDR > 2/10,000/d, U5DR > 4/10,000/d GAM > 30% 20%+ of HH c food consumption grossly inadequate (<< 2100 kcal/p/d) Livelihood assets complete loss

Source: IPC Global Partners © 2012. Used with permission of FAO-UN on behalf of IPC Global Partnership.

4.   Therapy

IPC Phase 2 needs livelihood support.

IPC Phase 3+ needs above plus nutritional support.

Table 8.3.13
Nutritional Support of Malnourished Population

Nutritional Status	Therapy
Mild acute	Adequate general ration
Moderate acute (GAM > 10%)	Above + supplementary feeding or community therapeutic care
Severe acute (SAM > 2%)	Therapeutic feeding, community therapeutic care, or hospitalization

General Food Distribution (GFD)

2100 kcal/p/d requires 12 kg food/p/mo or $\approx$ 15 kg food/p/mo in logistics pipeline.
Ration—WFP commonly aims for 50% ration in settings where resources are limited.
Cost—$1000/MT Title II bulk food from US sources

Preventive Intervention (for populations on edge of frank malnutrition)

Targeted—see SFP below

Community Management of Acute Malnutrition (CMAM)

4 Components:
Stabilization Center (SC)
> admission criteria: age 6–59 mo, SAM (MUAC < 11.5 cm, WHZ <−3, or edema), anorexia, or severe medical complications
> treatment: F75, F100, IVF, ABX
> discharge criteria: appetite recovered, medical complication improved, pitting edema decreased, and clinically well

Outpatient Therapeutic Program (OTP)
> admission criteria: age 6–59 mo, SAM (MUAC <11.5 cm), appetite intact, and no severe medical complications
> treatment: RUTF (e.g. Plumpy'Nut® nutritionally = F100)
> discharge criteria: 15% weight gain (from entry weight), no bilateral pitting edema ×2 wks, and 2 mo minimum observation/treatment period

Supplementary Feeding Program (SFP)
> blanket—all HH in geographically targeted catchment area (e.g. where IPC 3+ and GAM > 15% or 10–14% with aggravating factors)
> targeted—some HH in catchment area (e.g. where GAM 10–14% or 5–9% with aggravating factors); U5 and pregnant or lactating women vs. U5 alone vs. U2 alone depending on resources available and challenges with case finding)
> overall programmatic target—50% coverage for SAM in rural areas (Sphere); 30% coverage for MAM in rural areas
> admission criteria:
>> pedes: age 6–59 mo, MUAC <12.5 cm, with appetite, discharged from OTP, no severe medical complications
>> pregnant & lactating: MUAC <21.0 cm, and 2nd–3rd trimester or with infant <6 mo
> treatment: RUSF as dry rations e.g. Plumpy'Sup®, CSB, CSB + (supercereal), CSB ++ (supercereal +)
>> NB   CSB may also be cooked on-site as in emergency school feeding.
> discharge criteria (pedes): weight gain, MUAC >12.5 cm, time in program > 2 months

Community Outreach with Mobile Brigades

Therapeutic Feeding Program

Admission criteria for U5: SAM (WHZ < −3, MUAC < 11.5 cm, or bilateral pitting edema)
Discharge criteria for U5: WHZ >−2.5, no edema, and clinically well (generally takes 4–6 weeks)
Treatment protocol (WHO, ICDDR)
> Shock   Severe dehydration: RL + D5, ½ strength Darrow's + D5,
>> or ½ NS + D5Dose: 100 cc/kg IV

Table 8.3.14
IV Therapy of Severe Dehydration

Age	Initial bolus	Balance
<1 year	30 cc/kg IV over 1 h	70 cc/kg IV over 5 h
>1 year	30 cc/kg IV over ½ h	70 cc/kg IV over 2 ½ h
If severely malnourished (WHO)	15 cc/kg IV over 1 h + ReSoMal 10 cc/kg by NGT	if improved after initial bolus, repeat 15 cc/kg IV over 1 h + ReSoMal 10 cc/kg/h PO/NGT × 10 h; if not improved after initial bolus, assume septic shock
If severely malnourished (ICDDR)	20 cc/kg IV over 1 h	10 cc/kg/h over 10 h + ORS 5–10 cc/kg PO after each loose stool

Dehydration

    Moderate dehydration (5–10%): ReSoMal PO or NGT

    With malnutrition: Dose 75–100 cc/kg PO/NGT over 12 h given as 5 cc/kg/half h × 4, then 5–10 cc/kg/h × 10 h (WHO)

    Without malnutrition: Dose 75–100 cc/kg PO over 4 h (if age > 1 yr) or over 6 h (if < age 1 yr) (ICDDR)

    NB   ICDDR does not use ReSoMal but prefers rice-based ORS for all patients with diarrhea

Feeding c̄ therapeutic milks—F75 (Phase 1), F100 (Phase 2)

    D10 or F75 for hypoglycemia; blankets/warmer for hypothermia

    3 Rx—ABX, mebendazole, antimalarial

    Adjuncts—vitamins A–D, minerals, measles vaccine, Fe (only in rehab phase)

    a. process indicators
        (1)   daily average weight gain at TFC: > 8 g/kg/p
    b. outcome indicators
        (1)   cure
        (2)   complications (~25% SAM will have medical complications)
        (3)   death (~25% SAM will die with good care, and 50% will die with mediocre care)

Table 8.3.15
Exit Indicators in Therapeutic Feeding Programs

Setting/reference		Exit indicator			
		Cure	Mortality	Default	Non-Response
TFC	Target (SPHERE)	>75%	<10%	<15%	
	Target (NGO)	>80%	<5%	<10%	
	Alert (NGO)	<50%	>15%	>25%	
SFC	Target (SPHERE)	>75%	<3%	<15%	
	Target (NGO)	>75%	<3%	<15%	<20%
	Alert (NGO)	<50%	>10%	>30%	>30%

C.   Micronutrient Deficiency

Table 8.3.16
Micronutrient Deficiency States

Micronutrients	Disease	Clinical Findings
Vitamins		
A	Avitamnosis A	night blindness, xerophthalmia, Bitot's spots, corneal ulcer/keratomalacia, corneal scars
B_1 (Thiamine)	Beri-beri	wet (acute)—congestive heart failure, anasarca; dry (chronic)—peripheral neuropathy (e.g. sensory Δs, wrist drop), weakness, weight loss, progressive ascending weakness (can't stand from a squat)
B_2 (Riboflavin)		cheilosis, angular stomatitis, glossitis
B_3 (Niacin)	Pellagra	dermatitis (sun-exposed areas e.g. Casal's necklace; tongue bright red), diarrhea, dementia, death (4 Ds)
B_9 (Folate)	Anemia	glossitis, others as per anemia below
C	Scurvy	gingivitis, dental loosening, petechiae, delayed wound healing
D	Rickets	bone-cartilage junctions enlarged at ribs (rachitic beads), wrists, & ankles; frontal bossing; sternal prominence; long bones bowed; joints with "splaying, cupping, & fraying"
Minerals		
I	Hypothyroid	goiter, cretinism (mental retardation, short stature, squint, deaf-mutism)
Zn	Zinc deficiency	diarrhea, delayed wound healing
Other Cofactors		
Fe	Anemia	fatigue, dyspnea, pallor, mental dullness (#1 nutritional disorder in the world)

VIII. CHEMICAL WEAPONS

A. Chemical Agents

Table 8.3.17
Chemical Agent Characteristics, Clinical Effects, and Treatments

		Chemical agents			
Agent	**Physical Characteristics**	**Systems Affected**	**Sx**	**Decon First Aid**	**Tx Antidote**
Blister Mustard (H, HD, HN)	oily light yellow-brown liquids with odor of garlic	eye—few hrs; resp & derm—2–24 h; **lethal in large doses**	red skin, blisters, eye burning, coughing	remove agent, S&W, flush with dilute bleach	none, supportive care
Blister Lewisite (L)	oily colorless liquid with odor of geraniums	derm—immediate pain; **lethal in large doses**	skin pain or irritation, eye burning, coughing	remove agent, S&W, flush with dilute bleach	BAL, supportive care
Blister Phosgene oxime (CX)	solid < 95° F but vaporizes	derm—immediate pain **lethal in large doses**	skin pain, wheals, eye burning, coughing	remove agent, S&W, flush with dilute bleach	none, supportive care
Blood Cyanide (AC)	rapid evaporating liquids with odor of bitter almonds; gas lighter than air	resp, heme—death in min; **highly lethal**	cherry red skin or lips, rapid respirations, dizziness, HA, seizures, death	usually none; leave area, aeration, S&W	amyl nitrite, Na thiosulfate
Blood Cyanogen Cl (CK)	rapid evaporating liquids with odor of bitter almonds; gas heavier than air	resp, heme—death in min; **highly lethal**	cherry red skin or lips, rapid respirations, dizziness, HA, seizures, death	usually none; leave area, aeration, S&W	amyl nitrite, Na thiosulfate
Choking Phosgene (CG)	rapid evaporating liquid with odor of mown hay	resp, derm—death in days; **lethal in large doses**	eye and resp irritation	leave area, aeration, s&w, eye irrigation	none, supportive care
Choking Chlorine (Cl)	gas at room temp	resp—death in days; **lethal in large doses**	eye & resp irritation, chest tightness, delayed pulm edema	leave area, aeration, S&W, eye irrigation	none, supportive care
Nerve Tabun (GA), Sarin (GB), Soman (GD)	colorless, odorless liquid; G agents less volatile than water	resp—seconds to minutes; derm—min to hrs; **highly lethal**	blurry vision, twitching, chest tightness, SOB, SLUDGE, brady, broncho-spasm, seizures	remove agent, S&W, flush with dilute bleach	atropine, 2-PAM
Nerve VX	slight yellow colored liquid at room temp; V agents as volatile as motor oil	resp—seconds to minutes; derm—min to hrs; **highly lethal**	blurry vision, twitching, chest tightness, SOB, SLUDGE, brady, bronchospasm, seizures	remove agent, S&W, flush with dilute bleach	atropine, 2-PAM
Riot control Tear gas (CS), Mace (CN)	gas at room temp	resp—seconds; non-lethal	eye & resp irritation	leave area, aeration, S&W, eye irrigation	none

BAL	British anti-Lewisite
2-PAM	2-pyridine aldoxime methyl chloride
S&W	soap and water
SLUDGE	salivation, lacrimation, urination, defecation, GI distress, emesis
SOB	shortness of breath

B. **Management of MCI from Suspected Chemical Weapons** (adapted from Domestic Preparedness Training [10])

Overarching rule: **all responders should wear personal protective equipment to avoid becoming a victim**.

Notification Phase (RAIN)

1. **R**ecognize a problem
   a. mass casualties
   b. syndromic casualty pattern
   c. dissemination device
   d. warning from perpetrator
   e. patient (host)—compelling symptoms
   f. agent—identifiable sights or smells
   g. environment—dead animals
2. **A**void
   a. distance—100 m from chemical attack, 300 m from explosion
   b. direction—upwind, upgrade, upstream
   c. 4 don'ts—don't become a victim, don't rush in, don't TEST (taste, eat, smell, touch), don't assume anything
3. **I**solate
   a. cordon off the area to extent possible
   b. isolate the casualties
4. **N**otify authorities
   a. informant
   b. agent released
   c. immediate morbidity and mortality
   d. signs and symptoms
   e. type of device/vehicle/container—specify sights, smells, sounds
   f. secondary disaster of fire or explosion
   g. wind direction, weather conditions
   h. witnesses
   i. lead responder
   j. actions taken
   k. actions forthcoming
   l. meeting place for responders
   m. follow-up contact (time, means, channel)

Response Phase

1. Site security
   a. position equipment upwind, upgrade, and upstream from incident site
   b. isolate the area including downwind vapor hazard area
   c. establish hot (ambient hazard), warm (contaminated victims), and cold (clean treatment) zones
2. Staff protection
   a. PPE for providers in the hot zone
   b. ICS to manage the incident
   c. SOPs to guide responder actions
3. Social controls (PINS)
   a. **P**reserve evidence
   b. **I**dentify the agent
   c. **N**eutralize contaminated areas
   d. **S**earch for secondary devices
4. Environmental and case management
   a. corral casualties and victims
   b. establish decontamination stations

    c. perform decontamination

    d. provide first aid—triage, treat, transport

Emergency Self-decontamination

1. Wet or blot (blotting for chemical contamination; wetting down for bio or nuclear contamination)
2. Strip off clothing
3. Flush the affected area with water or dilute bleach
4. Cover the affected area

C.   Implications for Disaster Management

1. Forensic
2. Clinical
3. Epidemiological
4. Pharmacological
5. Environmental
6. Social
7. Judicial
8. Political

IX.   EPI METHODS

A.   Study Types

1. Assessments and appraisals
2. Surveys
3. Surveillance
4. Screening

B.   Study Designs

1. Prospective
   - a. concurrent (cohort)
   - b. nonconcurrent (retrospective cohort or trohoc)
2. Retrospective, case control

Measures of association quantify the strength or magnitude of the association between the exposure and the health problem of interest. They are independent of the size of the study and may be thought of as best guess of the true degree of association in the source population. However, they give no indication of the association's reliability.

- cohort study—relative risk (RR) = riskexposed/riskunexposed
- in acute outbreaks, risk is represented by the attack rate (AR)
- case-control study—odds ratio (OR)
- no denominator with which to calculate an attack rate
- cross-sectional—prevalence ratio or prevalence odds ratio

C.   Survey Designs (see R Magnani [11], and F Checchi [12])

1. Census—complete enumeration of the entire population
2. Sample
   - a. probability sampling
     - (1) simple random sampling (SRS)
       It requires a complete enumeration of population N—names and locations of all persons or households (HH)—and sample size n
     - NB Much effort is necessary to conform to requirements of random sampling. It is easier to sample less often but take more specimens as a cluster. Unfortunately, it is recognized that individuals from a cluster often share characteristics which < the precision of the method.

(2)   systematic random sampling

It requires a complete enumeration of population N, and sample size n, to calculate the skip interval $k = N/n$.

(3)   stratified random sampling

It requires a population size N divided into groups or strata L, then SRS within each stratum. The method ensures over-sampling in under-represented groups. It yields separate estimates for each stratum at less cost. However, it requires extra info and has complicated analysis.

(4)   cluster sampling, cluster sample survey (CSS)

It is used when you don't have a complete enumeration N of all people in the area, and thus can't do random sampling; or when the area is too big to cover, and thus can't do systematic random sampling.

- What should be done to compensate for the bias induced when one samples clusters rather than individuals? Use 2n. Empiric data on association within clusters in smallpox immunization suggests doubling n. If $n = 96$, $2n = 192$.

- What is the minimum number of clusters that can be selected and still fulfill requirements of the theory on which binomial sampling is based? 30. Statistical theory demonstrates that ≥ 30 clusters help ensure cluster means have a normal distribution. The larger the number of clusters, the smaller the design effect (i.e. study efficiency improves, and the total number of study subjects needed will decrease). E.g. 40×20 ($n = 800$) will prove more accurate and efficient than 30×30 ($n = 900$). 50 clusters $\times$ 30 households will be more precise, but 30 clusters $\times$ 50 households may be more logistically feasible. Choice of cluster should be driven by what one team can complete in a day. 30×30 CSS leaves 7.5 min/HH/team, but 45×18 CSS leaves 15 min/HH/team. If a team can only measure 20 kids/day (which is common), then it's best to increase the number of smaller clusters.

- To permit an equal number of children to be selected from each of 30 clusters, 6 children would not achieve the necessary n. Therefore, 7 children are selected per cluster ($30 \times 7 = 210$).

b.   non-probability sampling

(1)   convenience

(2)   purposeful/judgment (most affected area, HHs, etc.)

(3)   quota

D.   **Bias** (see R Magnani [11], F Checchi [12], and SMART [13])

Systematic, non-sampling error which lowers accuracy of findings. It is usually not appreciated by the survey team. It is usually not apparent from the survey results. It cannot be arithmetically calculated or corrected. Its extent cannot be judged by readers of the report. Methods and materials must be explicit. Report authors must discuss possible sources of bias as limitations to their study. Accuracy depends on validity of findings. It is more important than precision (Section E), and bias should be prevented at all costs. Awareness of sources of bias is the first step in minimizing its impact on any study. As sample size increases, it is more difficult to control quality. More teams to train and supervise create higher risk of bias. It is better to have smaller sample size with less attendant precision but much less risk of bias.

1.   Selection bias—respondents are not representative of the population

a.   project bias—assessors work where a project may be conceptually familiar to them

b.   spatial/access bias—assessors work where access is easiest (roadside or "windshield" bias)

c.   refusal or non-response bias (self-selection) bias—subject nonparticipation may undermine representativeness of the sample

d.   survivor bias—assessments are conducted where households have disappeared due to family death or migration. Mortality rate is thereby underestimated. This bias is most likely where HH size is low, recall period is long, mortality is high, and clustering is present.

  e. class/ethnic bias—different social classes or ethnic groups are inadequately included if not excluded from the assessment. Local assessors may have ethnic bias, or the key informants may be drawn from one particular social class or ethnic group.

  f. season bias—assessments are conducted during harvest season or periods of weather when segments of the population may be under-represented

  g. time of day/schedule bias—assessments are conducted at a time of day when segments of the population may be under-represented

NB Items 2–3 below may also be grouped as information/measurement bias.

2. Interview bias

  a. interviewer bias

   (1) cultural bias—assessors cultural norms lead to incorrect assumptions about the interview subjects

   (2) mandate or specialty bias—assessors mandate or specialty blinds them to needs outside of that mandate or specialty. E.g., a shelter specialist may only assess shelter needs while neglecting livelihood or nutrition needs.

   (3) gender bias—assessors interview only one gender

   (4) language bias—assessors may have a limited spectrum of people with whom they can communicate

   (5) key informant bias—assessors may be partial to key informants who appear credible in ways meaningful to the assessors

   (6) information/political bias—assessors focus on information that confirms preconceived notions rather than pursue evidence of alternate beliefs

   (7) mistranslation

   (8) interviewer error—assessors write down answers incorrectly

  b. subject (response) bias

   (1) event recall bias—retrospective surveys only, esp. with recall periods > 1 yr

    (a) informants underreport remote events (e.g. neonatal deaths)

    (b) calendar bias—informants over report events within the recall period

   (2) event reporting bias

    (a) taboos—informants underreport taboo subjects (e.g. neonatal deaths)

    (b) lies—informants misinterpret surveys as registration activities and over report family members or underreport deaths to maintain assistance

    (c) political bias—informants present information that conforms to their political agenda

   (3) age heaping/digit preference—informants exhibit digit preference

3. Instrument/measurement bias—errors in design or use of instrument (e.g. questionnaire, lab equipment, etc.)

  a. random errors in measurement

  random errors in weight measurement, even if yielding equal numbers of high and low measurements, widen the distribution curve without altering the mean. Hence, the prevalence of malnutrition is overestimated. The effect is greater for severe malnutrition than for moderate malnutrition, and greater when prevalence is low than when it is high. The data distribution should be checked for normal distribution with an SD between 0.8 and 1.2 z scores. Improving the data quality thus appears to reduce the prevalence of malnutrition.

  b. systematic errors in measurement

  systematic errors in weight measurement, even if small (e.g. 30 g error in presence of clothing), may alter the mean, but also widen the distribution curve. Hence, the prevalence of malnutrition is overestimated. Systematic errors in height measurement, such as erroneous lengthboard, may alter the mean without altering the SD. If the measurement is too short, there will be > stunting, albeit < wasting. If the measurement is too long, there will be < stunting, albeit > wasting. A standardization test is routine before undertaking anthropometric surveys.

  NB Some scholars prefers terms "counted" and "calculated" to "measured" and "derived"

4. Data entry bias

5. Analytic bias

a. anchoring bias—focusing on one major piece of information
b. confirmation bias—favoring data which confirm underlying beliefs
c. familiarity bias—weighing familiar/understandable events and spokespersons more than unfamiliar ones
d. recency bias—weighing recent events more than remote ones
e. salience bias—weighing vivid events more than mundane ones
f. "time will tell" bias—collecting more data or letting time pass instead of making a hard decision

E. **Imprecision** (see R Magnani [11], F Checchi [12], and SMART [13])

Sampling, non-systematic error which lowers precision of findings and affects the level of certainty in extrapolating sampling estimates to the population's true value. It is always present, unavoidable, and a function of chance. Its magnitude depends on sample size, sampling statistics, prevalence of condition, and length of recall period. Precision refers to consistency of results obtained from repeated measurements.

1. Sample size
   What is the sample size n of a random sample of binomial variables needed to yield a result of specified accuracy and precision?
   $n = [(z^2pq)/d^2] \times$ design effect

   e.g. 1   n = first estimate of sample size

   z = confidence limits (accuracy), or normal deviate. Usually set at 95%

   ∴ z "score" = 1.96

   p = proportion of the target population with attribute p

   q = proportion of the population without attribute p = 1 – p. Usually set at 0.5 to maximize the n of a study having a result of specified accuracy and precision. If you knew p and q, you would not need to do a survey.

   d = confidence interval (precision). Usually set at +/− 10%

   ∴ d = .1

   design effect (see 2e below)

   $$n = \frac{(1.96)^2 (0.5)(0.5)}{(0.1)^2}$$

   n = 96

   e.g. 2   There is a population of 6000 where the expected disease rate is 12%. To measure the prevalence with precision of 2%, what sample size is required?

   $$n = \frac{(1.96)^2 (0.12)(0.88)}{(0.02)^2}$$

   n = 1014

   Once n is calculated, compare it to the size of the target population (N). If n < 10% of N, then use n as final sample size. If n > 10% of N, then recalculate the final sample size (n_f) by the following correction (a smaller sample size may be used).

   $$n_f = \frac{n}{1 + n/N}$$

   $n_f = 1014/1.169$

   $n_f = 867$

   NB   n to calculate the mean weight may be much smaller than n to calculate the prevalence of malnourished outliers (120 vs. 900).

2. Sampling statistics and error measurement
   a. malnutrition prevalence or death rate
      The higher the prevalence (or death rate), the lesser the precision (higher d) available through a fixed sample size. (This is a consequence of the formula.) 10% GAM is a common trigger for intervention. But, SMART discourages use of this because high survey precision is needed (narrow CI).
      ∴ Choose highest expected prevalence or rate—tends to > n.
      NB At levels of malnutrition and mortality generally found in emergencies, precision has much greater effect on sample size than suspected prevalence of malnutrition or death rate. n is related to d^2. E.g., if the malnutrition rate estimate is 10%, and assuming a design effect of 2:
      • survey statistic with a CI of +/− 3% requires $n = 768$
      • survey statistic with a CI of +/− 2% requires $n = 1729$
      As rule of thumb, prevalence (%)/2 approximates the range of appropriate CI. E.g. malnutrition prevalence of 20% calls for a precision of +/− 5% (range of 10%). It's generally unfeasible to achieve precision greater than +/− 3%.

Table 8.3.18
Malnutrition Prevalance and Study Precision

Expected Prevalence	Precision
5–10%	+/− 3%
10–15%	+/− 3.5%
15–20%	+/− 4%
20%+	+/− 5%

   b. standard deviation (SD, σ).
      the degree to which individuals within the sample differ from the sample mean (μ); unaffected by sample size
   c. standard error (SE = SD/$\sqrt{n}$)
      Standard deviation of the sampling distribution of a statistic; decreases with larger sample sizes as estimate of the population mean improves, thus a lower SE is more precise
      (1) standard error of the mean (SEM) is standard deviation of a sample mean's estimate of a population's true mean; an estimate of how close to the population's true mean the sample mean appears to be.
      (2) relative standard error (RSE)—SEM/μ expressed as %
          • SE of 700 g on weight mean of 70 kg = RSE of 1%
          • SE of 1400 g on weight mean of 70 kg = RSE of 2%
   d. confidence interval (CI = μ ± z (SE))
      The margin of error around a point estimate. For normally distributed data, the CI yields the range in which a parameter is 95% likely to be found. A convention for reporting such data would be: "the most probable estimate of the parameter is X, and we are 95% confident the parameter lies somewhere between Y and Z [bounds of the CI]" (paraphrased from Checchi, 2005).
      NB In general, the lower the prevalence (or death rate), the greater the precision (lower d) needed to detect it and any subsequent changes in it. (This is intuitive.) Overall, there is no benchmark for precision. Increasing precision (decreasing d) slightly can dramatically increase n. +/− 0.4 deaths/10,000/d is a practical limit in precision of mortality surveys.
      ∴ Choose widest acceptable CI—tends to < n.
   e. design effect (D_{eff} = variance$_{study\ design}$/variance$_{simple\ random\ sample}$)
      a measure of the (in)efficiency of a cluster sample survey compared to that of a simple random sample. If $D_{eff} > 1$, but the analysis treats it as a SRS, then the confidence interval is inappropriately narrowed, and a test for differences is more likely to produce a positive result (Type 1 error).
      • If each child in a cluster had an unrelated probability of immunization, the precision of the sample estimate would match that of a simple random sample in which 210 children were chosen. $D_{eff} = 1$. However, this is generally not the case.

- If each child in a cluster had an identical probability of immunization, the precision of the sample estimate would match that of a simple random sample in which 30 children were chosen. D_{eff} = cluster size of 7.

NB   Focal phenomena create clustering of findings which increase the D_{eff}.

Table 8.3.19
Design Effect of Various Phenomena

Magnitude	D_{eff}	Examples
Low	< 2.5 (gen 1.5, trends up to 2.0 in large studies)	malnutrition (wasting, stunting, underweight), anemia, EPI, mortality studies
Moderate	2.5–7.0	diarrhea, ARI, malnutrition c edema (kwashiorkor)
High	7.0–10.0	measles immunization
Very high	>10	access to potable water, latrines, mortality from violence (Iraq surveys had D_{eff} of 19)

∴   Choose largest D_{eff}—tends to > n.

3.   Length of recall period
   a.   The shorter the recall period, the more accurate the mortality estimate (more distant events are more likely to be forgotten).
   b.   The longer the recall period, the more precise the mortality estimate for a fixed sample size. The "sample" is effectively the number of person-days. For a fixed level of precision, the length of the recall period is inversely related to number of study subjects needed. If you cannot increase the sample size, you must increase the recall period.

F.   Confounding

Confounders are extraneous variables that correlate with both dependent and independent variables of interest (e.g. both the exposure of interest and the outcome of interest), are unevenly distributed across the levels of exposure, but are not causally linked to exposure and outcome. Age and sex are the most common confounders. Hence, the importance of matching in intervention and control groups.

G.   Validity

1.   Study validity
   a.   internal—capacity of the study to yield sound conclusions for the study population after considering **bias, imprecision, and confounding** (see D-F above)
   b.   external—generalizability beyond the study population (ill-advised)
2.   Measurement validity
   a.   criterion validity
      (1)   concurrent—sensitivity/specificity or correlation with a gold standard
      (2)   predictive—ability to predict an event
   b.   face validity—common sense
   c.   content validity—all relevant elements of a composite variable are included
   d.   construct validity (usually for a new measure)—extent to which the measure corresponds to theoretical concepts (constructs)
   e.   consensual validity—extent to which experts agree the measure is valid
   ∴   Strength of evidence: face validity, criterion validity > content, construct, consensual validity. In absence of validity, a measurement may be embraced for its reliability (below).

H.   Rates

1.   Death rates—calculated incidence of death expressed per 10,000 p/d or per 1000 p/mo; data collected by retrospective surveys (e.g. 3 month period) to gauge severity of public health emergency particularly where sudden events lead to spike in mortality
   a.   CDR—crude death rate

b. ASDR—age-specific death rate (e.g. U5DR or death rate of children 0–5 yr) during a studied time interval (written as $_5M_0$ or 0-5DR); age of study cohort, e.g. 0–5 yr, should not be confused with study time intervals

Table 8.3.20
Representative Death Rates

Situation	CDR	0-5DR
Baseline in developing countries	<< 1	1
Emergency under control	<1	<2
Serious trouble	1–2	2–4
Emergency out of control	>2	>4
Catastrophe	>4	

2. Mortality rates—calculated probability of dying before a specified age expressed per 1000 live births; data collected by national health authorities in periodic (annual) demographic surveys to reflect ongoing health status
   a. CMR—calculated probability of mortality in given population for specific time
   b. IMR—calculated probability of a live borne child dying before 1 yr
   c. U5MR—calculated probability of a live borne child dying before 5 yr

NB MR ≠ DR. E.g. CMR ≠ CDR, U5MR ≠ U5DR. Different rates measure different things and are not directly comparable. However, MRs may be converted into DRs by the following: CDR or U5DR (deaths/10,000/d) = - ln(1-p/1000) × 5.47 where p = CMR or U5MR (deaths/1000 live births). However, this has little field utility.

NB MMR—maternal mortality ratio has different units in numerators (maternal deaths) and denominators (live births), thus is a ratio, not a rate

I. **Reliability/Reproducibility**

1. Stability—inter/intra-observer variation
   a. discrete variables—kappa coefficient
   b. continuous variables—correlation coefficient
2. Internal consistency—correlation among all items in the measure
3. Tests of reliability—Cronbach's alpha, Kuder-Richardson, split halves

J. **Conclusions**

1. Interpolation
   The application of study findings to an entire population from which the sample was drawn. If the survey was well-conducted, the results may be considered representative of the entire population. This is scientifically justified. However a CI should accompany any parameter estimate of that population.
2. Extrapolation
   The extension of study findings to a population or period which was not represented in the sample. It works by association—if 2 populations appear to be experiencing similar conditions, the morbidity/mortality experience of one may be imputed to the other. This is not scientifically justified, but is often done where data are insufficient or impossible to collect.

K. **Major Criteria in Evaluating a Health Intervention**

1. Does it < mortality?
2. Does it < morbidity?
3. Does it enhance the health system?
4. Does it lower cost?

References

1. Declaration of Alma-Ata. International Conference on Primary Health Care, Alma-Ata, USSR, 6–12 September 1978. Available from http://www.who.int/publications/almaata_declaration_en.pdf?ua=1.

2. Walsh, J., & Warren, K. (1979). Selective primary health care—An interim strategy for disease control in developing countries. *New England Journal of Medicine, 301*, 967–974.

3. US Centers for Disease Control and Prevention (1999). Ten great public health achievements—United States, 1900–1999. *Morbidity and Mortality Weekly Report, 48*(12), 241–244.

4. US Centers for Disease Control and Prevention. (2011). Ten great public health achievements—United States, 2001–2010. *Morbidity and Mortality Weekly Report, 60*(19), 619–623.

5. Mara, D., & Feachem, R. G. (1999). Water and excreta-related diseases: unitary environmental classification. *Journal of Environmental Engineering, 125*(4), 334–339.

6. Feachem, R. G. (1983). Infections related to water and excreta: the health dimension of the decade. In: *Water supply and sanitation in developing countries*. London: Institution of Water Engineers and Scientists.

7. World Health Organization. Global database on child growth and malnutrition. Available from https://www.who.int/nutgrowthdb/about/introduction/en/index5.html.

8. IPC Global Partners. (2016). Addendum to IPC Technical Manual Version 2.0. *Tools and procedures for classification of acute malnutrition.* Rome: IPC Global Partnership, 2016. p 14.

9. IPC Global Partners. (2012) Integrated Food Security Phase Classification Technical Manual Version 2.0. *Evidence and standards for better food security decisions* (p. 32). Rome: FAO-UN on behalf of IPC Global Partners.

10. NBC Domestic Preparedness Training Hospital Provider Course. Undated. Curriculum available from the Center for Domestic Preparedness, Anniston AL, http://cdp.dhs.gov/.

11. Magnani, R. (1997). *Sampling guide*. Washington, DC: FANTA, 1997. Available from www.fantaprojet.org.

12. Checchi, F., & Roberts, L. (2005). *Interpreting and using mortality data in humanitarian emergencies—a primer for non-epidemiologists.* Humanitarian Practice Network, Network Paper No 52. London: Overseas Development Institute, Sept 2005.

13. Standardized Monitoring & Assessment of Relief & Transitions (SMART). (2006). Measuring mortality, nutritional status, and food security in crisis situations: SMART methodology. v1. April 2006. Available from http://pdf.usaid.gov/pdf_docs/Pnadi428.pdf.

Annex 8.4
TROPICAL MEDICINE

Glossary

abd	abdomen
ABX	antibiotics
ACP	asymptomatic cyst passer
ACT	artemisinin-based combination therapy
AF	acid-fast (e.g. Ziehl-Neelsen)
AFP	acute flaccid paralysis
Ag	antigen
aggl	agglutination
AHF	acute hepatic failure
AIDS	acquired immunodeficiency syndrome
AR	attack rate
ARDS	acute respiratory distress syndrome
ARF	acute renal failure
ARI	acute respiratory infection
ART	antiretroviral therapy
Aus	Australia
AVB	atrioventricular block
BAL	bronchoalveolar lavage
BC	blood culture
BM	bone marrow
BW (A, B)	biological weapon, biological warfare (threat class)
Bx	biopsy
c	century; with
C	centigrade; chills
CA	Central America
Ca	cancer
CE	complex emergency
CFR	case fatality ratio
CHF	congestive heart failure
CI	chronic illnesses
CMI	cell-mediated immunity
CMP	cardiomyopathy
CNS	central nervous system
CP	complications
CSF	cerebrospinal fluid
CT	chemotherapy; cholera toxin; computed tomography
d	day(s)
D	diarrhea
DAA	direct-acting antivirals
DC	developing country
DDx	differential diagnosis
DF	dengue fever
DIC	disseminated intravascular coagulation
DOTS	directly observed therapy short course
DRC	Democratic Republic of the Congo
Dx	diagnosis
E	east, eastern
EAEC	enteroadherent *E. coli*
EHEC	enterohemorrhagic *E. coli*
EIEC	enteroinvasive *E. coli*
ELISA	enzyme-linked immunosorbent assay
EM	erythema migrans
ENL	erythema nodosum leprosum
ETEC	enterotoxigenic *E. coli*
Eur	Europe
exts	extremities
F	female; fever
FAR	fever, arthritis, and rash
FO	fecal-oral
FQ	fluoroquinolone
FSU	former Soviet Union
FTT	failure to thrive
FUO	fever of unknown origin
GB	gall bladder
GI	gastrointestinal
GIB	gastrointestinal bleed
H2H	human-to-human (transmission)
HA	headache

HAV	hepatitis A virus
HB	heart block; hepatitis B
HBIG	hepatitis B immunoglobulin
HBV	hepatitis B virus
HCC	hepatocellular carcinoma
HD	heart disease
HeAn	hemolytic anemia
hemor	hemorrhage
HF	hemorrhagic fever
HIV	human immunodeficiency virus
HM	hepatomegaly
HSM	hepatosplenomegaly
HSV	herpes simplex virus
HTN	hypertension
HUS	hemolytic-uremic syndrome
HZ	herpes zoster
I	incidence
IC	industrialized country
ICP	immunocompromised person
ID	infectious disease
ID_{50}	median infectious dose
IDU	injecting drug user
IE	infective endocarditis
IFA	immunofluorescence assay
IG	immune (serum) globulin
JH	Jarisch-Herxheimer (reaction)
LA	Latin America (Central America + South America)
LBRF	louse-borne relapsing fever
LBTF	louse-borne typhus fever
LBW	low birth weight
LE	lower extremity
LF	Lassa fever
LGV	lymphogranuloma venereum
LN	lymph node, lymphadenopathy
Lx	laboratory
M	male
MB	multibacillary
MDR	multidrug resistant
ME	Middle East
MM	mucous membranes
MODS	multiple organ dysfunction syndrome
MS	mental status
N	nausea; north, northern
NA	North America
NAf	North Africa
NFI	nerve function impairment
NH	northern hemisphere
NL	normal
NV	nausea and vomiting
OD	opportunistic disease
OI	opportunistic infection
org	pathological organism
p	after
P	prevalence
PB	paucibacillary
PCN	penicillin
PCR	polymerase chain reaction
PEP	post-exposure prophylaxis
perf	perforation
PGL	persistent generalized lymphadenopathy
PMN	polymorphonuclear leukocyte
PNG	Papua New Guinea
PS	peripheral blood smear
Pt	patient
PUD	peptic ulcer disease
Px	physical exam
RBBB	right bundle branch block
RDT	rapid diagnostic test
RHZE	rifampicin + isoniazid + pyrazinamide + ethambutol
RTPCR	reverse transcriptase polymerase chain reaction
RUQ	right upper quadrant
Rx	drug therapy
s	without
S	south, southern
SA	South America
SAFE	surgery, antibiotics, facial cleanliness, environmental improvement
SAM	severe acute malnutrition

SBE	subacute bacterial endocarditis
SC	stool culture
SD1	S. dysenteriae type 1
SE	southeast
SM	splenomegaly
SSA	sub-Saharan Africa
SSD	sickle cell disease
S/Sx	signs and symptoms
STEC	shiga toxin-producing E. coli
STI	sexually transmitted infection
Sx	symptoms
Sz	seizure
TB	tuberculosis
TIG	tetanus immune globulin
TMP/SMZ	trimethoprim + sulfamethoxazole
TPE	tropical pulmonary eosinophilia
Tx	treatment
U5	under 5 year-old
UC	urine culture
UE	upper extremity
US	ultrasound
UTI	urinary tract infection
V	vomiting
VBD	vector-borne disease
VE	viral encephalitis
VHF	viral hemorrhagic fever
VL	visceral leishmaniasis
W	west, western
wk	week
YF	yellow fever
Δ	change in
//	similar to

Pathophysiology

Why does this person from this place get this disease at this time?

Person — Think of new exposure for Pts from non-endemic or developed areas. Think of breakdown in immunity for Pts from endemic or undeveloped areas. For systemic infection, infective dose is a function of immunity and innoculum.

immunity relates to host and may be altered by congenital, acquired, or iatrogenic causes

innoculum relates to infectious organism and the environment

Place — Think geographic medicine.

Time — Think seasonality. Malaria is classic:

- Holo-endemic areas (e.g. Congo) have an intense level of malaria transmission year-round. Epidemics don't occur unless displacement brings in non-immune populations. Infection may be asymptomatic. Effective partial immunity develops in adults which enables clinical tolerance of infection and protects against serious episodes. Mortality is highest in pedes U5 and pregnant women.

- Hyper-endemic areas (e.g. W. Africa) have an intense but unstable level of transmission in seasonal peaks when the climatic conditions are favorable. Epidemics occur. Infection is generally symptomatic. Partial immunity fails to develop. Mortality occurs across all age groups.

- Hypo-endemic areas (e.g. Thai-Burmese border) have a low level of transmission year-round. Epidemics occur. Infection is generally symptomatic. Partial immunity fails to develop. Mortality occurs across all age groups.

Sx — Think differential diagnosis (below).

Differential Diagnosis or Special Considerations in Common Presentations

Etiological summary   trauma, vessel, neoplasm, infection, drugs, toxins, congenital, metabolic, endocrine, nutrition, connective tissue diseases (autoimmune), psyc

Diarrhea

watery (secretory, small intestine)

viruses, *E. coli* (ETEC, EAEC), campylobacter, salmonella, vibrio, bacillus, C. *perfringens*, enteric protozoa except entamoeba

NB   giardia, cryptospordium often yield frothy D due to gut malabsorption

bloody (inflammatory, large intestine)

E. coli (EHEC or STEC e.g. O157:H7, EIEC), campylobacter, salmonella, shigella, C. *difficile*, yersinia; entamoeba

Dyspnea

hantavirus pulmonary syndrome and pneumonic plague present similarly and are co-endemic

Fever < 7 d

PMNs >   focal bacterial infections, lepto, amoeba (liver abscess), borrelia, sepsis (non-typhi salmonella, pneumococcus, staph, strep, meningococcus)

PMNs < or NL   rickettsia, malaria, typhoid, viruses

s localizing signs   sepsis (non-typhi salmonella, pneumococci, staph, strep, meningococcus), malaria, UTI, typhoid, HIV

Lx: malaria smear, BC, UC, serology

rash/hemorrhage   as for fever s focal bacterial infections or amoeba

petechial rash   meningococcal sepsis, IE, DIC, Henoch-Schonlein purpura, VHF

jaundice   bacteria/parasite (coxiella, lepto, malaria, sepsis); SSD; viruses (YF, hepatitis); worms (ascaris, echinococcus, liver flukes)

Fever > 7 d

PMNs >   leprosy (erythema nodosum leprosum), amoeba (liver abscess), borrelia, deep sepsis

Eos >   tissue nematodes, zoonotic nematodes, strongyloides > other gut nematodes c heart-lung migration, cestodes (excluding gut tapeworms), trematodes

PMNs NL   brucella, chronic meningococcal sepsis, SBE, syphilis, TB (localized), toxo, tryps

PMNs <   brucella, HIV, malaria, TB (disseminated), typhoid, VL

NB   fever + Δ vital functions = emergency

fever + any 2 = potentially lethal lesion (e.g. fever + jaundice + acute renal failure)

borrelia // lepto in acute fevers; coxiella // brucella in chronic fevers

Hepatomegaly

hepatitis, hepatoma, hepatic abscess, hydatid, schisto, TB, malaria

Jaundice

prehepatic   malaria, sepsis, hemolysis, hemoglobinopathy

hepatic   viral hepatitis, YF, Q fever, lepto, drugs

post-hepatic   gallstones, choledochocarcinoma, hydatid in biliary tree, ascariasis in biliary tree, liver flukes

Neuro signs unexplained TB, HIV and OIs, syphilis, Lyme disease, Whipple's disease, brain abscess

Paralysis

flaccid   Guillain-Barre syndrome (immune mediated), polio (anterior horn infection)

spastic   trauma, vascular, neoplasm, infection—HIV/HTLV, abscess, TB, subacute combined degeneration

Splenomegaly—massive

congestive   SSD, schisto

reactive   malaria

infiltrative   amyloid, VL, lymphoma, leukemia

combined

Splenomegaly—moderate

above + differential diagnosis for F > 7 d c̄ PMNs < or NL

STI—bubo

ulcer   chancroid, granuloma inguinale

no ulcer   LGV

no STD   plague, filariasis, LE infection

STI—ulcer

single, painless   1° syphilis (s̄ LN), LGV (transient, c̄ bubo), granuloma inguinale (persistent and progressive c̄ pseudobuboes)

granuloma diseases start with one painless ulcer, but develop painful bubos

superinfection of painless lesion, TB

single, painful   2° syphilis

mult, painless

mult, painful   herpes (often c̄ systemic Sx & LN), chancroid (c̄ bubo)

BW syndromes

   many BW agents initially present as flu-like syndrome (F, C, HA, malaise, myalgia)

influenza

pulmonary   anthrax*, plague, tularemia, Q fever, melioidosis, hantavirus

jaundice   HA

encephalitis   VE, Q fever

rash, cutaneous   smallpox*, tularemia, typhus fever

septicemia/shock   anthrax*, plague, typhus fever, VHF

occult death

*   not further characterized as tropical disease in Tables 8.4.1 and 8.4.2 below

Vectors and Intermediate Hosts

Vector—comes to you (not necessarily required for development of the organism)

mosquitoes and ticks transmit the most types of infectious pathogens

Aedes transmit all mosquito-vectored VHF

Intermediate hosts—you come to the intermediate host (required for development of the organism)

intestinal nematodes have none

all trematodes + 1 zoonotic nematode require snails

Management Keys

Know the local epidemiology

Leading U5 causes of death worldwide—LRI (15%), prematurity (15%), birth asphyxia (11%), diarrhea (9%), malaria (7%), neonatal sepsis (7%)

Leading ID causes of death worldwide—LRI, diarrhea, HIV/AIDS, TB, malaria, measles, meningitis

Know the golden rules of infectious diseases (abstracted from A Yung [1] and used with permission).

1. Rigors are always important—serious bacterial infections are the most likely cause.
2. Severe muscle pain may be a symptom of sepsis even without fever.
3. Elderly patients with sepsis may be afebrile. In elderly patients, fever is rarely caused by a viral infection.
4. Septic patients who are hypothermic have a worse prognosis than those with high fever. Treat as a medical emergency.
5. Fever in a postoperative patient is usually related to the surgical procedure (e.g. pneumonia, UTI, wound, or deep infection).
6. Fever with jaundice is rarely due to viral hepatitis. Think liver abscess, cholangitis, etc.
7. The rash of early meningococcal infection may resemble a viral rash.
8. Generalized rashes involving the palms and soles may be due to drugs, viral infections, rickettsial infections, or syphilis.
9. All febrile travelers in or returned from a malaria infected area must have malaria excluded.
10. Disseminated TB must be suspected in all elderly patients with fever and multisystem disease who have been in an area with endemic TB.
11. Septic arthritis may be present even in a joint which is mobile.
12. Back pain with fever may be caused by vertebral osteomyelitis or an epidural abscess.
13. A patient may have more than one infection requiring treatment (e.g. malaria and typhoid), especially if they are elderly, immunosuppressed, or have travelled.
14. Always remember common infections, not just opportunistic infections, in AIDS patients with a fever.

Understand morbidity multipliers.

measles, malnutrition, and TB/HIV

Understand occult co-morbidities.

For any undifferentiated illness, even in infants, think of HIV, TB, syphilis, and sarcoid.

For any child, think of malaria, hookworm, & anemia; malarial anemia usually in pedes <3 year-old, hookworm anemia usually in pedes >3 year-old.

For any ICP, think of TB, VL, histoplasmosis, strongyloides. Must treat early.

DDx Failure to thrive without F in infants is worked up like F without localizing signs.

Watch for clinical mimics—malaria presenting as pneumonia or diarrhea in pedes; VL presenting as malaria in adults; lepto presenting as mild DF (esp in DF endemic areas where the Pt has mild onset of illness, worsening course, and no rash but jaundice after a week).

Tx Do basic things well, use equipment you understand, teach others, delegate.

Table 8.4.1a
Tropical Infectious Diseases—Vector-borne and Zoonotic

Vectors [Reservoir]	Organism	Group/Name — Fever, Arthritis, & Rash (FAR)	Clinical FAR	Clinical CNS	Clinical VHF	Clinical H2H	Misc	Annual Incidence or Prevalence	Deaths/year or CFR Rx, Vaccine
			acute Sx over 2–6 d—F, C, HA, back pain, arthralgia, mac-pap rash, desquamation; recovery over 2–3 wks				incubation < 3 wk; Lx—serology, ELISA, PCR; H2H—none		
Mosquitoes (F)									
Aedes	Alphavirus	Chikungunya Virus Disease (Kimakonde verb—to be contorted)	+				epidemic polyarthritis (favors wrists, hands, ankles, feet)	SSA, S & SE Asia, Caribbean	very rare; no vaccine
Anopheles [humans]	Alphavirus	O'nyong-nyong	+				epidemic polyarthritis	SSA	0
Aedes, Culex	Alphavirus	Ross River Fever	+				epidemic polyarthritis	Australia	0
Culex	Alphavirus	Sindbis Virus Disease (Ockelbo disease, Pogosta disease)	+				flu-like illness over 5d; CP of persisting arthritis	1-100s foci worldwide not NA, LA	0
Aedes aegypti, albopictus [humans—urban; monkeys—rural]	Flavivirus (4 serotypes) BW (A)	Dengue Fever (DF) (breakbone fever)	+	+			severe disease c F, C, retroorbital HA, back pain, myalgia, arthralgia, morbilli-form rash; CP of DHF	1-100,000,000 apparent 300,000,000 inapparent #1 viral VBD Asia, LA, SSA; rainy season	<1% vaccine in trial
Culex	Flavivirus BW (B)	West Nile Fever (WNF)	+	+			mild disease c F, malaise, HA, myalgia, anorexia, NV, rash → CNS (1%)	Africa, ME, Eur, NA, CA; early fall in NH	c CNS, 25% c FAR, 0% no vaccine
Aedes	Flavivirus	Zika Fever (from Zika Forest in Uganda)	+			STI	generally mild disease c F, malaise, HA, arthralgia, rash; neonatal microcephaly if contracted early in utero	Africa, Asia, Polynesia, SA	0 no vaccine
Sandflies (F)									
Phlebotomus	Bunyavirus	Sandfly Fever (phlebotomus fever, 3-day fever, pappataci fever)	+					S Europe, N Africa, E Mediterranean to N India	very rare
Phlebotomus	Rhabdovirus	Vesicular Stomatitis Virus (vesicular stomatitis fever)	+	+					very rare

Vector [Reservoir]	Virus (Family)	Disease					Clinical features	Distribution / Epidemiology	Mortality / Vaccine
Ticks (M & F)									
Dermacentor (wood tick)	Reovirus	Colorado Tick Fever (CTF) (mountain tick fever)	+				Biphasic illness over 6 d; rare CP of Δ CNS, VHF	W NA; summer	very rare no vaccine
		Viral Encephalitis (VE)	most infections asymptomatic; severe infections c F, HA, Δ MS, meningeal signs		+		incubation < 3 wk Lx—serology, ELISA, PCR H2H—Nipah		
Mosquitoes (F)									
Culiseta, Aedes [birds]	Alphavirus **BW (B)**	Eastern Equine E (EEE)		+			often severe	rare E NA, CA, SA	25–50% esp pedes vaccine for horses, but not humans
Culex, Culiseta [birds]	Alphavirus **BW (B)**	Western Equine E (WEE)		+			milder than EEE	rare W NA, CA, SA	5% vaccine for horses, but not humans
Aedes, Culex, et al [rodents, birds, horses]	Alphavirus **BW (B)**	Venezuelan Equine E (VEE)	+	+				large epidemics SA (esp Venezuela), CA, NA	<1% vaccine for horses, but not humans
Aedes [squirrels, lagomorphs]	Bunyavirus (serogroup c La Crosse E) **BW (B)**	California E		+				1-100 esp pedes W NA; summer, fall	< 1% no vaccine
Culex [water fowl, pigs]	Flavivirus **BW (B)**	Japanese E (JE)		+			99+% s Sx; 50% of survivors c neuro disability	70,000 esp pedes E Asia, S Asia, W Pacific	10,000 esp U5 20–30% vaccine
Culex [water fowl]	Flavivirus	Murray Valley E (MVE) (Australian E)		+			99%+ s Sx; 40% of survivors c neuro disability	Australia, PNG; summer monsoon season	25% no vaccine
Culex [birds]	Flavivirus **BW (B)**	St. Louis E (SLE)		+				NA, CA; summer, fall	5-15% no vaccine
Ticks (M & F)									
Ixodes [wild rodents]	Flavivirus (3 subtypes— European, Siberian, Far-eastern)	Tick-borne E (TBE)		+			biphasic illness—febrile phase c flu-like Sx → neuro phase c Δ CNS	I-5000 Eur, FSU, Asia; summer, fall esp rural & recreational areas	1–2% vaccine
[Mammals]									
horses, fruit bats	Hendra Virus	Hendra Virus Disease		+			pneumonia early	Australia	50% vaccine for horses, but not humans
pigs, fruit bats via urine or saliva contaminated fruits	Nipah Virus	Nipah Virus Disease		+		+	flu-like Sx initially	S Asia	50% vaccine for primates, but not humans

Vector / Reservoir	Virus	Disease			Clinical	Diagnosis	Epidemiology	Tx / Mortality
Dogs, foxes, coyotes, skunks, raccoons, bats (infectious saliva)	Rabies Virus	Rabies (hydrophobia)			F, HA → 2 syndromes: encephalitic (furious) rabies (80%)—intermittent agitation & terror // mania alt c lucid intervals, autonomic hyperactivity, bulbar spasm to water (hydrophobia), spasticity, sz → **death in days**; paralytic rabies (20%)—ascending sensorimotor AFP, fasciculation, paraparesis, bulbar paralysis s hydrophobia → **death in wks**	serology; skin Bx for IFA	worldwide mostly in developing countries; 50% of people bitten by infected animal contract disease	50,000 s Tx 100% first aid of bites: scrub with soap and water vaccine
		Viral Hemorrhagic Fever (VHF)			F, malaise, HA, conjunctivitis, pharyngitis, myalgia, arthralgia, rash (morbilliform to petechial); CP of Δ vasc perm, bleeding, shock, ARF, AHF, MODS	incubation <3 wk Lx—serology, ELISA, PCR H2H—many but only from Pt c Sx		
Mosquitoes (F)								
Aedes, Culex, et al [livestock via inoculation or inhalation; abortion storm heralds human transmission risk]	Bunyavirus	Rift Valley Fever (RVF)	+	+	5% c Δ CNS or HF		sporadic epidemics NAf, SSA, ME	overall < 1% VHF 50% ribavirin; vaccine for animals, but not humans
BW (A)								
Aedes aegypti, albopictus [humans—urban; monkeys—rural]	Flavivirus (4 serotypes)	Dengue HF/Dengue Shock Syndrome (DHF/DSS)	+	+	biphasic illness— F phase then cap leak c 4 clinical classes		1-500,000 pedes < 15 S, SE Asia, W Pacific; rainy season	25,000 s Tx > 20% c Tx 2% no vaccine
BW (A)								
Aedes aegypti, et al [humans—urban; monkeys—rural]	Flavivirus	Yellow Fever (YF)	+		F, C, HA, NV, jaundice; CP (20%) of AHF, GIB, ARF		1-200,000 endemic SSA (90% cases) > sporadic LA not Asia	30,000 endemic 10% sporadic 50% vaccine
Ticks (M & F)								
Hyalomma via tick bite or direct contact with blood from infected animal or human	Bunyavirus	Congo-Crimea HF (CCHF)	+	+	flu-like Sx—F, HA, eye pain, myalgias, abd pain, hepatitis; CP of hemor **rapidly fatal (2 wks) s Tx**		Central, S Asia, Africa; esp butchers, shepherds	20-50% ribavirin; no vaccine
BW (A)								
Haemaphysalis [rodents, shrews]	Flavivirus	Kyasanur Forest Disease (monkey fever)	+	+	flu-like Sx—F, HA, myalgias; CP of hemor in biphasic illness		1-500 India	3-5%
Dermacentor	Flavivirus	Omsk HF	+	+	flu-like Sx—F, C, HA, myalgias, palatal rash, cervical LN; CP of hemor, Δ CNS		FSU esp Siberia	1-3%

[Mammals]

Reservoir / Transmission	Agent	Disease			Clinical	Epidemiology	Treatment / Vaccine
Calomys (rodents) via aerosols from urine, saliva, or stool, or food contamination	Arenavirus **BW (A)**	Argentine HF (Junin)	+	+	VHF // LF, but 1/3 of untreated cases become c hemor and neuro signs	I-100 C Argentina; Mar–Apr; farm workers at corn harvest	s Tx 20% c Tx <2% vaccine
Calomys (rodents) via aerosols from urine, saliva, or stool, or food contamination	Arenavirus **BW (A)**	Bolivian HF (Machupo) (black typhus)	+	+ (low)	VHF Sx + low back pain	Bolivia	s Tx 20%
rodents suspected via aerosols from urine, saliva, or stool, or food contamination	Arenavirus	Brazilian HF (Sabia)	+	+	VHF // LF, but 1/3 of untreated cases become c hemor and neuro signs	Brazil	no vaccine
Sigmodon, et al (cotton rat, cane mouse) via aerosols from urine, saliva, or stool, or food contamination	Arenavirus **BW (A)**	Venezuelan HF (Guanarito)	+	+	VHF // LF, but 1/3 of untreated cases become c hemor and neuro signs	W Venezuela; Nov–Jan	s Tx >30% no vaccine
Mastomys, et al (rodents) via aerosols or direct contact with stool or urine	Arenavirus **BW (A)**	Lassa Fever (LF)	+	+ (high)	most s Sx; VHF Sx in 4 phases: F, malaise, fatigue (1–3 d); HA, sore throat, myalgia, DNV, cough (4–7 d); edema, bleeding (20% of Pt c Sx), Δ CNS (7+ d); coma (14 d); deafness common in survivors	100,000–300,000 W SSA; Jan–May; most common VHF c H2H in travelers	5000; 2–20% ribavirin; experimental vaccine
Mastomys (rodents)	Arenavirus **BW (A)**	Lujo HF	+	+	VHF Sx	<10 in history S Africa, Zambia	s Tx 80%
Apodemus, et al (field mice) via bites or aerosols from urine, saliva, or stool	Bunyavirus (Hantavirus is 1 of 5 genera) **BW (A)**	Hemorrhagic Fever with Renal Syndrome (HFRS) (Korean hemorrhagic fever from Hantan River area in S Korea)	+		5 phases: F, HA, malaise, back pain, NV, conj injection, rash (3–7 d); ↓ BP due to hemor (1–3 d); oliguria (3–7 d); diuresis (wks); recovery (months)	E Asia, Eur, NA, SA; late fall, early winter	c Tx 5–15% ribavirin; experimental vaccine
Peromyscus, et al (deer mice) as above	Bunyavirus (Hantavirus is 1 of 5 genera) **BW (A)**	Hantavirus Pulmonary Syndrome (hantavirus ARDS)		+ (low)	cardiopulmonary syndrome	as above; only Andes variant capable of H2H transmission	c Tx 30–40% no vaccine
? fruit bats → gorillas, duikers via saliva contaminated dropped fruits	Filovirus (5 types of Ebola; Sudan strain mildest) **BW (A)**	Ebola-Marburg Diseases (EHF, African HF)	+	+	VHF Sx + DNV; VHF CP (50% of Pt c hemor); **rapidly fatal s Tx**	SSA	Ebola 60–90% Marburg 30% experimental vaccine

Table 8.4.1b
Tropical Infectious Diseases—Vector-Borne and Zoonotic

Vectors [Reservoir]	Organism	Non-viral Diseases			Annual Incidence or Prevalence	Deaths/year or CFR Rx
		Name	Clinical	Lab Diagnosis		
Bugs (M & F)						
Triatoma (cone-nosed, kissing bugs) via direct contact with vector feces, food contamination, or congenital [humans in chronic disease]	*Trypanosoma cruzi*	American Trypanosomiasis (Chagas' disease)	acute—chagoma, F, LN, HSM; chronic (25%)—HD (CMP, RBBB, CHF), megacolon	amastigotes in tissue Bx; tryps in stained PS (rare); serology	I-300,000 P-10,000,000 LA (3rd most common VBD p malaria & DF)	11,000 rare acutely nifurtimox
Fleas (M & F)						
Xenopsylla via feces [rodents, feral cats, opossums]	*Rickettsia typhi*	Typhus Fever (FBTF) (endemic, murine)	// LBTF but milder	serology	worldwide; warm climates esp summer-fall	1–5% doxycycline
Xenopsylla, Pulex via regurgitation, direct contact c org from infected HH pets [rodents] ... BW (A)	*Yersinia pestis*	Plague	bubonic—sudden onset F, C, extreme malaise, myalgia, tender LN at site of inoculation (bubo); CP of sepsis, pneumonia (pneumonic plague), meningitis, DIC; 10–25% of plague cases have primary septicemia; **yes H2H; rapidly fatal s Tx**	bacteria in smear, gram stain	I-< 2500 worldwide foci; Africa esp DRC	bubonic s Tx 50% pneumonic s Tx 100% streptomycin, gentamycin, doxycycline
Flies (gen F)						
Phlebotomus, et al (sandflies, F)	*Leishmania*	Cutaneous Leishmaniasis (CL) (Baghdad boil, Delhi boil, rose of Jericho)	papule → nodule → painless ulcer occas c nodular lymphangitis, LN; CP of mucosal involvement (espundia) in New World disease	amastigotes in stained slit skin smears; culture; Leishmanin test	I-1,000,000 worldwide foci; most in SA, Mediterranean, & ME-central Asia	rare sodium stibogluconate (New World only)
Phlebotomus, et al (sandflies, F) [various mammals]	*Leishmania donovani et al* (Old World), *chagasi* (New World)	Visceral Leishmaniasis (VL) (kala-azar = black fever)	most s Sx; F, LN, massive HSM → cirrhosis, pancytopenia, dark skin at head & mouth (kala-azar); some c F, malaise, cough, D (// malaria); post-K-A dermal leish (PKDL) c diffuse papules & nodules at mouth, face, & trunk	amastigotes in spleen > liver > BM > LN aspirate; serology	I-200–400k worldwide foci; 90% in rural (sub) tropics of Brazil, Ethiopia, India, Somalia, S Sudan, Sudan	20–40,000 10% sodium stibogluconate

Vector	Organism	Disease	Clinical features	Diagnosis	Epidemiology	Tx
Chrysops (deerflies, F)	*Loa loa*	Loiasis (Calabar swelling, African eyeworm)	most s Sx; migratory Calabar swellings, pruritis, myalgia; CP of F, HA, meningism	micro filariae in stained PS of noon spec	P-13,000,000 tropical SSA rainforest	0 DEC
Culicoides (biting midges, F)	*Mansonella*	Mansonelliasis	most s Sx; transient itch, HA, arthralgia	micro filariae in stained PS	SSA, LA	0 albendazole rarely needed
Simulium (blackflies, F)	*Onchocerca*	Onchocerciasis (river blindness)	most s Sx; SC nodules, itch, rash (sowda, lizard skin, leopard skin), blindness	micro filariae in skin Bx; if non-Dx, DEC challenge	P-18,000,000 300k blind SSA >> LA riverine areas	0 ivermectin + albendazole
Glossina (tsetse flies, M & F) [humans—*Tbg*; cattle, game—*Tbr*]	*Trypanosoma brucei gambiense, rhodesiense*	African Trypanosomiasis (sleeping sickness)	chancre (occas c hemor) → hemolymphatic stage—F, HA, local & occipital LN, SM → CNS stage— psyc Δs, sleep Δs, tremor, ataxia; *Tbr* >> *Tbg*	tryps in stained PS, lymph, CSF; serology	1-500,000 W SSA *Tbg* E SSA *Tbr*	400,000 s Tx 100% s CNS suramin c CNS melarsoprol

Lice (M & F)

Vector	Organism	Disease	Clinical features	Diagnosis	Epidemiology	Tx
Pediculus humanus (body, clothing lice) via feces, not directly via bite [humans] heavy clothing + poor sanitation = lice proliferation	*Bartonella quintana*	Trench Fever (Quintana fever)	F, malaise, HA, SM, shin pain, rash	BC; serology	foci in Central Asia, LA, E & N Africa	0 doxycycline × 5 d; wash clothes at 50 °C or leave unworn × 1 wk
Pediculus humanus (body, clothing lice) via feces, not directly via bite [humans] heavy clothing + poor sanitation = lice proliferation	*Borrelia recurrentis*	Relapsing Fever (LBRF) (epidemic, louse-borne)	F 2–9 d alt s F 2–4 d c 1–3 relapses; assoc c HA, myalgia, NV, HSM, jaundice, petechial rash, Δ CNS; CP of nephritis, meningitis, myocarditis; **may be rapidly fatal s Tx**	orgs in stained or darkfield PS	foci in cold, rural, highland, temperate areas of Asia, E Africa, SA	s Tx 10% doxycycline × 5 d (JH in 90%); wash clothes at 50 °C or leave unworn × 1 wk
Pediculus humanus corporis (body lice) via feces, not directly via bite [humans] heavy clothing + poor sanitation = lice proliferation	*Rickettsia prowazekii* **BW (B)**	Typhus Fever (LBTF) (epidemic, classic, jail fever, red louse disease) vector color indicative as bacteria multiply in gut & lyse epithelium → blood enters body cavity turning louse red; recrudescence years later = Brill-Zinsser disease	malaise, myalgia 1–3 d → high F, C, HA, Δ CNS —delirium, stupor, coma, prostration, centrifugal rash d5 (central mac-pap → peripheral petechiae & purpura s face, palms, or soles), vasculitis c symmetric digital gangrene, strokes, shock, MODS; **rapidly fatal s Tx**: recrudescence gen short & mild	serology—Weil-Felix reaction, IFA (gold standard)	foci in cold, rural, highland, temperate areas of Asia (Russia), E Africa (Great Lakes, Ethiopia), SA (Peru); winter-spring; massive deaths in wars, famines, & migrations	s Tx 10–60% esp > 60 y/o c Tx < 5% doxycycline × 5 d (200 mg ×1 dose in epidemics); wash clothes at 50 °C or leave unworn × 1 wk

Vector	Organism	Disease	Clinical	Diagnosis	Epidemiology	Tx / Mortality
Mites (M & F larvae)						
Leptotrombidium (trombiculid larval mites or chiggers) via saliva [rodents]	*Orientia* (prev *Rickettsia*) *tsutsugamushi*	Scrub Typhus (MBTF) (mite typhus, Tsutsugamushi fever)	painless ulcer, eschar (distinguishes case from DDx of malaria, typhoid) → // LBTF + conjunctivitis, LN, HSM → vasculitis c DIC, ARF, MODS; **fatal s Tx** but lower mortality than LBTF	serology—Weil-Felix reaction, IFA (gold standard)	foci in scrub areas of S, SE Asia, Pacific islands; monsoon season	s Tx 1–30% gen < LBTF doxycycline
Liponyssoides	*Rickettsia*	Rickettsial Pox (vesicular rickettsiosis)	papule, LN; F, vesicular rash (s palms, soles)	serology	E NA, Central Asia	rare doxycycline
Mosquitoes (F)						
Anopheles	*Plasmodium falciparum, vivax, ovale, malariae*	Malaria (swamp fever)	*Pf* CP of cerebral malaria, ARDS, ARF (adults); **rapidly fatal s Tx**	orgs in stained PS, RDT	1-200,000,000 #1 parasitic disease SSA, Asia, LA	438,000 90% in SSA nearly all U5 quinine, ACT
Culex, Anopheles, Aedes, et al	*Wuchereria bancrofti, Brugia malayi, timori*	Filariasis (lymphatic filariasis)	most s Sx; *Wb* c recurrent F, LN, retrograde lymphangitis, lymphedema, TPE; CP of elephantiasis (limbs, breasts, genitals); *Bm, Bt* // *Wb* but F worse, CP only in distal exts	micro filariae in stained PS of midnight spec, skin Bx; serology —Ag detection	P-110,000,000 S, SE Asia, SSA, LA P-13,000,000 S, SE Asia	0 albendazole + DEC or ivermectin (in oncho areas)
Ticks (M & F)						
Ixodes (hard ticks in Ixodidae family e.g. deer ticks)	*Babesia*	Babesiosis	most s Sx; F, C, malaise, myalgia, jaundice from HeAn, s rash	orgs in stained PS	worldwide foci	clindamycin + quinine
Ixodes (hard ticks in Ixodidae family e.g. deer ticks)	*Borrelia burgdorferi*	Lyme Disease	red papule → 1st stage (1–4 wks)—EM: 2nd stage (1–6 months)—F, HA, malaise, LN, EM (s palms & soles), neuro Sx (esp bilat Bell's), cardiac Sx (esp AVB), arthropathy (esp knees); 3rd stage (years)—episodic oligoarthritis, chronic myocarditis, polyneuropathy	serology is inaccurate	NA, Eur, Asia; summer	doxycycline
Borrelia duttoni, et al (soft ticks in Argasidae family)	*Ornithodoros*	Relapsing Fever (TBRF) (endemic, tick-borne)	// LBRF but milder (< HSM, jaundice, rash) c more relapses & longer course	orgs in stained or darkfield PS	SSA (Somalia), ME, S Asia, NA, SA	s Tx < 2–10% doxycycline JH in 40%
Amblyomma, Ixodes (hard ticks in Ixodidae family)	*Ehrlichia*	Ehrlichiosis	F, C, HA, malaise, myalgia, sore throat s rash	serology	USA, Japan not tropics	< 2% doxycycline
Dermacentor, et al (hard ticks in Ixodidae family e.g. wood ticks, dog ticks) via tick bite, aerosols from infected hosts, food contamination [rodents, lagomorphs] **BW (A)**	*Francisella*	Tularemia (rabbit fever)	vector bite → local ulcer, regional LN; inhalation → F, C, HA, fatigue, pneumonia or sepsis; ingestion → pharyngitis, abd pain, DNV; **no H2H**	serology at 2 wks		rare s Tx 5–10% gentamycin

Vector	Organism	Disease	Clinical features	Dx	Geography	Tx/mortality
Amblyomma (hard ticks in Ixodidae family)	*Rickettsia africae*	African Tick Bite Fever	multiple painless eschars, lymphangitis, LN, subtle rash // TBTF	serology	SSA; people on safari	0 doxycycline
Rhipicephalus sp. (hard ticks in Ixodidae family e.g. brown dog ticks)	*Rickettsia conorii* complex (multiple sero-types)	Tick-borne Typhus Fever (TBTF) (Mediterranean tick fever or spotted fever, boutonneuse fever, tick typhus of Kenya, Crimea, India, Israel)	painless button eschar, LN, peripheral mac-pap rash d4 (palms, soles, & face)	serology	Africa, India, Mediterranean	3–30% doxycycline
Dermacentor, et al (hard ticks in Ixodidae family e.g. dog ticks, wood ticks)	*Rickettsia rickettsii*	Rocky Mtn Spotted Fever (RMSF) (NA tick typhus, Sao Paolo fever, Tobia fever)	F, C, malaise, HA, myalgia, centripetal rash d5 (pink macules on palms, soles, & face → central petechiae)	serology	E NA, LA; summer	s Tx 15–25% c Tx 3–5% doxycycline
> 40 tick species	none—neurotoxin	Tick Paralysis	ascending, lower motor neuron paralysis c paresthesis → progressive c bulbar & resp paralysis	none—Dx is based on finding the tick; DDx Guillain-Barre	worldwide foci; most in W NA, E Australia	rare esp pedes < 10 supportive Tx

Table 8.4.2
Tropical Infectious Diseases—Non-vector-borne

Hosts [Intermediate] Mechanism	Organism	Group/name	Diseases — Clinical	Diseases — Lab Diagnosis	Annual Incidence or Prevalence	Deaths/year or CFR Rx
			Bacteria			
	Actinomyces	Actinomycosis	induration & draining sinuses in jaw, thorax (DDx fungi)	orgs in gram stain	worldwide sporadic	ampicillin
cats	*Bartonella henselae*	Cat-scratch Disease	regional LN (10% suppurate); atypical presentations (5%) c lung or liver lesions, encephalitis, FUO	IFA; Bx	worldwide	none azithromycin or none
cattle, pigs, goats, sheep	*Brucella abortus, melitensis, suis* **BW (B)**	Brucellosis (undulant fever, Malta fever)	recurrent F, C, night sweats, lethargy, HA, arthralgia, visceral μ abscesses, wt loss; CP of osteoarthritis, orchitis, endocarditis, meningitis	BC, BM culture; serology; PCR	worldwide	s Tx 2% rifampicin + doxycycline
environmental saprophyte [none—soil reservoir; animals may contract illness, but org is not zoonosis]	*Burkholderia pseudomallei* **BW (B)**	Melioidosis (Whitmore's disease, first described in Myanmar)	most s Sx; bacteremia (60%) c sepsis, multiple abscesses, or typhoidal syndrome c ICPs or CIs; localized infection (40%) esp in lung (may look //`TB), liver, spleen, skin → late reactivations	BC, UC, pus culture; serology	SE Asia, N Aus, SSA, LA; esp ICPs; rainy season	ceftazidime; chloro + cotri + doxycycline
	Chlamydia	Trachoma	conjunctival folliculitis → intense inflammation → scarring → trichiasis → corneal opacity → scarring → blindness	orgs in epithelial cells of conj swab	P-150,000,000 2m blind worldwide dry areas	SAFE c azithromycin, tetracycline ointment
	Clostridium	Tetanus	onset 1 wk p injury; neonate— weakness, floppiness, irritability, inability to feed, spasms; adult—trismus, local & generalized spasms (4 prognostic classes)	none—Dx is clinical	I-1,000,000 pedes I-200,000	10–90% PCN + TIG
	Coryne-bacterium	Diphtheria	F, toxicity, tonsillopharyngitis c pseudomembrane & bleeding points, LN, neck edema; painful, cutaneous ulceration c palsy; CP of airway obstruction, myocarditis, HB			non-cutaneous 5–10% procaine PCN + antitoxin
sheep, cattle, goats, cats, dogs via airborne	*Coxiella burnetii* **BW (B)**	Q Fever (query fever)	acute—F, C, malaise, HA, atypical pneumonia; chronic (<1%)—FUO, granulomatous hepatitis c jaundice, endocarditis	serology	worldwide hot, dusty areas esp ranchers, livestock farmers	<2% doxycycline, FQ
cattle, other ruminants	*Escherichia coli* (6 pathotypes— ETEC, EHEC, EIEC, etc.) **BW (B)**	Gastroenteritis (travelers diarrhea, shiga toxin-producing *E. coli*)	acute DNV; dysentery if EHEC, EIEC; CP (5–10%) of HUS from EHEC O157:H7	SC	I-200,000,000 ETEC	380,000 ETEC mostly U5 in DCs no vaccine

	Organism	Disease	Clinical features	Dx	Epidemiology	Treatment/Notes
rodents, pigs, cattle, dogs, raccoons via skin or MM	*Leptospira*	Leptospirosis (hemorrhagic jaundice, mud fever, ricefield fever, canecutter's disease, swineherd disease, Weil's disease)	anicteric syndrome (90%) (due to bacteremia)—F, C, HA, DNV, cough, conjunctivitis, rash, myalgia (lumbar & calf), malaise; myocardial, renal, liver disease (10%) → icteric syndrome (1%) (Weil's disease)—anicteric syndrome + HSM, deep jaundice, rash (orange skin), HeAn, purpura, GIB, HUS, ARF, AHF	serology	worldwide tropics c fresh water rivers, floods, or rainy season; esp farming, abattoir, sewerage workers; riverine tourists	Weil's 10% doxycycline, PCN
	Neisseria meningitides (serogroups A, B, C W, Y)	Meningococcal Disease	sepsis, meningitis, petechial rash; **rapidly fatal s Tx**	orgs in CSF gram stain; BC, CSF culture	1-500,000 esp U5 worldwide; dry season epidemics of group A in SSA	30-60,000 c Tx 10% ceftriaxone
	Salmonella enterica var Paratyphi (pathotypes A, B, C)	Paratyphoid Fever	// typhoid F but milder—F, NVD (occas dysentery) c 10 d course; CP of bacteremia → bone, joints, GB, other organs (esp in SSD, HIV)	BC, SC	1-<< typhoid F	<< typhoid F FQ, ceftriaxone
	Salmonella enterica var Typhi **BW (B)**	Typhoid Fever (enteric fever, typhus abdominalis—confused c epidemic typhus thru 18th c)	sustained or remittent F, C, malaise, fatigue, relative brady, HA, cough, myalgia, anorexia, N, abd pain, constipation, D, HSM, rose spots; CP of lower GIB (10%) & bowel perf (3%) from Peyer's patches, encephalopathy, meningitis, ARF, abscess	BC > SC wk 1 SC > BC wk 2+ UC, BM culture if above NG; Widal poor test but used in DCs	1-27,000,000 epidemic AR 6% P-2-5% infected chronically S Asia >> Africa	600,000 s Tx 10-20% c Tx < 1% highest CFR U5 FQ, ceftriaxone
	Shigella (4 species—*S. dysenteriae* type 1 (SD1) most severe, esp in emerg settings; *S. flexneri* most common in DCs; *S. sonnei* most common in ICs; *S. sonnei* & *S. boydii* c mild D) **BW (B)**	Shigellosis (bacillary dysentery)	F, NVD (initially watery, then small volume dysentery), anorexia, low abd pain, cramps, tenesmus, rectal prolapse (pedes); 25% will not have dysentery, but when present, it can last wks-months; CP (esp in SD1) of hypoglycemia, sepsis, encephalopathy, toxic megacolon, GI perf, HUS	SC, BC ID_{50} for SD1 = 10 SD1 (Shiga bacillus) produces Shiga toxin causing severest disease, longest duration of illness, higher ABX resistance, and highest CFR	1-175,000,000 esp U5, malnourished; endemic in Africa & Asia	1,000,000 mostly U5 s Tx 20% FQ

Organism	Disease	Clinical	Dx/Lab	Epidemiology	Treatment
Streptococcus	Rheumatic Fever	major manifestations—carditis (mitral > aortic), polyarthritis (large joints), chorea, ery marginatum, or subcut nodules; minor manifestations—arthralgia, fever	serology e.g. ASO titer. Dx is clinical (2 major or 1 major + 2 minor) supported by Lx	I-300,000 P-15,000,000 developing countries; winter-spring esp adolescents	225,000 benzathine PCN
Treponema pallidum pertenue	Yaws	3 phases—papilloma → frambesial lesions (wks–months); widespread esp palms & soles (months); destruction of skin & bone at exts (10%+ of Pts) (5 years)		P-2,500,000 tropics; esp pedes	benzathine PCN, azithromycin
Vibrio cholerae (O1 & O139 serogroups cause epidemics. O1 El Tor is cause of current (7th) pandemic. Other serogroups cause individual ill-ness.) **BW (B)**	Cholera	afebrile DNV c acute onset of profuse, painless, ricewater stools. No clinical differences between epidemic strains.	SC ID_{50} = 100,000+ 1st test is agglutination c O1 & O139 antisera. O1 serogroup divided into Inaba & Ogawa serotypes, plus classical & El Tor biotypes. All strains tested for CT—strains s CT do not cause epidemics.	I-2,800,000 worldwide; epidemic AR: 5% (refugees c malnut); 2% (rural underserved in non-endemic areas); 1% (WHO typical estimate of overall disease burden); 0.6% (endemic areas c poor sanitation)	100,000 s Tx 50% in severe disease c Tx <1%
Sexually Transmitted			**Bacteria and HSV**		
Chlamydia trachomatis	Lymphogranuloma Venereum (LGV) (tropical bubo)	single, small, painless, transient genital ulcer → suppurative inguinal & pelvic LN (M c inguinal buboes, F c proctitis); CP of lymphedema, rectal stricture	IFA, PCR, culture of LN aspirate; serology	worldwide esp tropics & subtropics	rare doxycycline, erythromycin x 3 wks
Haemophilus ducreyi	Chancroid (soft chancre)	single or multiple deep, painful, necrotic, soft ulcers → painful, suppurative LN	culture, IFA, PCR of exudate; serology	worldwide esp inner city; M > F	0 ciprofloxacin × 3 d
Herpes Simplex virus (HSV)	Herpes Simplex	multiple painful vesiculo-pustular lesions → ulcers → systemic Sx c nonsuppurative inguinal LN → resolution	Dx gen clinical; Tzanck prep, viral culture of lesion	worldwide	0 acyclovir
Klebsiella (prev *Calymmato-bacterium*) *granulomatis*	Granuloma Inguinale (donovanosis)	indurated papule → painless, beefy red ulcer c rolled edges → progressive ulceration & scarring c destruction of genitals → heme seeding to viscera & bone	orgs in stained granulation tissue smear, Bx; PCR	tropics & subtopics esp India, PNG, Caribbean	rare doxycycline, erythromycin × 3 wks

| *Treponema pallidum pallidum* | Syphilis (lues) | 1°— single, painless, firm chancre s LN (3 wks); 2°—mac-pap rash including palms & soles, generalized LN (6 wks); 3°—gummas (5 years), aortitis (10 years), meningitis (15 years). Pregnancy → still-birth (25%), neonatal death (15%), surviving syphilitic infant (40%) | serology | 12,000,000 worldwide | benzathine PCN |
| *Treponema pallidum pallidum* | Syphilis, congenital, early congenital | congenital—LBW, feeding difficulty, bullous rash, jaundice, HSM; early congenital—NL at birth, but develops FTT, rash (3 months) // 2° syph c desquamation of palms & soles, saddle nose, nasal discharge, HSM | serology | developing countries | benzathine PCN |

Mycobacteria

Organism	Disease	Clinical features	Diagnosis	Epidemiology	Treatment
Mycobacterium leprae	Leprosy (Hansen's disease)	hypopigmented/red skin patches c̄ ↓/absent sensation (no itch or sweat) (≤ 5 patches = PB, > 5 patches = MB), peripheral nerve thickening; evolution of asymmetric tuberculoid disease → symmetric lepromatous disease; early CP of Type 1 reactions (skin and nerve inflammation), Type 2 reactions (ENL, F, malaise), silent NFI; late CP of iritis, osteitis, loss of digits	orgs in AF stained slit skin smears ranging from PB to MB	P-650,000 S, SE Asia rural tropics	rifampicin + dapsone + clofazimine + steroids (if CP)
Mycobacterium tuberculosis	Tuberculosis (TB, consumption)	F, night sweats, wt loss, pulm Sx (85%), extrapulm Sx (15%)—LN (25%), pleurisy (25%), GU (15%), military (10%), bone (10%), CNS (5%), peritoneum (5%)	orgs in AF stained sputum, body fluid, or tissue Bx; miliary orgs in liver Bx > transbronchial Bx > BM	I-9,000,000 MDR 500,000 P-17,000,000 infected 2 billion disease risk: s HIV 5–10% over lifetime; c HIV 10%/year	1,400,000 430,000 HIV+ 50% die/year RHZE via DOTS
Mycobacterium ulcerans	Buruli Ulcer	painless, firm papule, nodule, or plaque (LE > UE) → ulcer c undermined edge → non-healing & extending	orgs in AF stained smear	worldwide tropics, SE Aus; esp pedes	rifampicin + adjunct ABX; debridement or excision if wide ulcer

Fungi

Organism	Disease	Clinical	Diagnosis	Geography	Frequency / Treatment
Subcutaneous					
Madurella, Pseudallescheria, et al	Mycetoma (maduromycosis, Madura foot)	painless, chronic subcut swelling, suppuration, & sinus tracts on extremities, esp foot; osteo	org clusters (granules) in smear, histology	N Africa (Sudan), S Asia, CA; esp barefoot	rare; miconazole
Phialophora, Fonsecaea, et al	Chromomycosis (chromoblastomycosis, dermatitis verrucosa)	dark-pigmented, warty, ulcerated, & pruritic plaques on LE extending to contiguous tissues over years	orgs in tissue Bx or scrapings; Bx culture	tropical LA, SSA; agric workers esp barefoot	rare; itraconazole
Sporothrix	Sporotrichosis	nodules → painless ulcer (DDx CL, anthrax) → lymphocutaneous (70%) c nodular tracks on cordlike lymphatics	culture of tissue Bx or pus; orgs rare on smear	worldwide; esp farmers & gardeners	rare; itraconazole
Systemic					
Endemic Respiratory					
Blastomyces	Blastomycosis (Gilchrist disease)	F, cough, pneumonia → chronic pulm disease → secondary spread c red papules, ulcers on face & distal exts	orgs in unstained sputum smears	worldwide; uncommon & sporadic	itraconazole, amphotericin
Coccidioides	Coccidioidomycosis (San Joaquin fever, desert fever)	F, C, cough; rarely body abscesses in subcut tissues	orgs in sputum smear, fluid, Bx	arid USA, LA; uncommon	high in disseminated disease; fluconazole, amphotericin
Histoplasma capsulatum	Histoplasmosis	5 syndromes: no Sx; acute pulm; acute disseminated (F, LN, HSM, BM suppression); chronic disseminated; chronic pulmonary disease // TB c cavitation	orgs in stained smears of body fluids	worldwide foci in LA, USA, Africa, Asia, Aus	itraconazole, amphotericin
Histoplasma capsulatum var duboisii	Histoplasmosis Duboisii (African histoplasmosis)	subacute, focal granuloma on skin, bone → secondary spread to skin, bone, LN, viscera	orgs in stained smear of granuloma, tissue Bx	Africa	itraconazole, amphotericin
Paracoccidioides	Paracoccidioidomycosis (S American blastomycosis)	pneumonia c patchy infiltrates → mucosal ulcerations, LN; visceral involvement	orgs in sputum smear, Bx; culture	tropical LA; esp agric workers	itraconazole, amphotericin

	Opportunistic Systemic				
Aspergillus	Aspergillosis	allergic bronchopulmonary aspergillosis; pulm aspergilloma (fungus ball); cold skin abscesses; invasive end organ effects in brain, kidneys	orgs in histology; culture	worldwide; uncommon & sporadic ICPs	itraconazole
Candida	Candidiasis	F, end organ effects	orgs in histology; culture	worldwide; ICPs	fluconazole amphotericin
Cryptococcus	Cryptococcosis	subacute-chronic meningitis esp in ICP; pneumonia	orgs in stained CSF; serology	worldwide; ICPs	fluconazole amphotericin
Pneumocystis jirovecii (prev *carinii*)	Pneumocystis Pneumonia (PCP) (plasma-cell pneumonia)	pneumonia in ICP	orgs in stained sputum, BAL, or lung Bx	worldwide; ICPs	TMP/SMZ
Rhizopus, et al (Mucoraceae)	Mucormycosis	nasal or paranasal infection → craniofacial necrosis; blood vessel thrombosis c infarction of lung, gut	orgs in tissue Bx; Bx culture	worldwide; ICPs	amphotericin

Helminths

Nematodes

Intestinal Nematodes

Host / Transmission	Genus	Disease	Clinical	Diagnosis	Epidemiology	Treatment
humans via FO [none—geohelminth]	Ascaris (roundworm)	Ascariasis	most s Sx; F, dry cough, wheeze (Loeffler's syndrome); intestinal worms rarely noted; colicky abd pain, bowel obstruction, appendicitis, pancreatitis	ova or worms in stool, sputum	P-1.5 billion tropics; esp pedes	mebendazole, albendazole
humans via FO [none]	Enterobius (threadworm, pinworm)	Enterobiasis	most s Sx; perianal itch, anorexia, D	ova on scotch tape swab (uncommon in stool)	P-350,000,000 esp pedes	mebendazole, albendazole
humans via skin of LE [none—geohelminth]	Ancylostoma, Necator (hookworm)	Ancylostomiasis, Necatoriasis	most s Sx; ground itch, cutaneous larva migrans (esp c dog & cat hookworms), dry cough (// Loeffler's), abd pain, D, hypochromic anemia	ova in stool (larvae in old specs)	P-900,000,000 women on agric plantation using nightsoil	50–60,000 mebendazole, albendazole
humans via skin of LE [none—geohelminth]	Strongyloides	Strongyloidiasis	triad of urticarial rash, abd pain (// PUD), D; also larva currens, dry cough (// Loeffler's), dysentery; CP of hyperinfection syndrome c foul D, malabsorption, bowel perf, sepsis, encephalitis	larvae in stool (ova uncommon unless D); duodenal aspirate; serology	P-60,000,000 co-existing c hookworm	albendazole, ivermectin preferred
humans via FO [none—geohelminth]	Trichuris (whipworm)	Trichuriasis	most s Sx; abd pain, chronic dysentery, rectal bleeding & prolapse, anemia, malnutrition (trichuris dysentery syndrome)	ova in stool; adult worm on sigmoidoscopy	P-500,000,000 tropics; esp pedes	rare mebendazole, albendazole

Filarial/Tissue Nematodes

Host / Transmission	Genus	Disease	Clinical	Diagnosis	Epidemiology	Treatment
	Loa loa	see vector table—flies				
	Mansonella	see vector table—flies				
	Onchocerca	see vector table—flies				
	Wuchereria, Brugia	see vector table—mosquitoes				

Zoonotic Nematodes

Host / Transmission	Genus	Disease	Clinical	Diagnosis	Epidemiology	Treatment
dogs, cats	Ancylostoma (dog, cat hookworm)	Cutaneous Larva Migrans (creeping eruption)	reticulated subcutaneous track on foot or buttock	none		albendazole, ivermectin
rodents [snails]	Angiostrongylus	Angiostrongyliasis (eosinophilic meningitis, visceral larva migrans)	meningitis, eosinophilia	often none; Hx of eating raw snails + meningitis + eos in PS, CSF; orgs in granuloma Bx	Asia-Pacific, LA tropics & subtropics	mebendazole

Organism	Disease	Host [reservoir/vector]	S/Sx	Dx	Geography / Prevalence	Tx
Anisakis	Anisakiasis (visceral larva migrans)	[marine fish]	abd pain, NV, enteric abscesses, malaise	orgs on endos-copy; tissue Bx; serology	Japan, Asia-Pacific, Scandinavia	excision
Dracunculus (Guinea worm)	Dracunculiasis	humans [none]	blister on leg/foot, ulcer; emergence of worm	none	P-100,000,000 SSA c dry Climate	extraction +/- ivermectin
Gnathostoma	Gnathostomiasis (visceral larva migrans)	dogs, cats [freshwater fish]	abd pain, NV, abd abscesses, malaise	orgs in granuloma Bx; serology	SE Asia	albendazole
Onchocerca (prev *Capillaria*)	Onchocerciasis (intestinal onchocerciasis)	[freshwater fish]	intermittent D, abd pain, malabsorption (protein losing), wt loss	ova or larvae in stool	Philippines, Thailand	rare but rapid metronidazole
Toxocara canis, cati (dog, cat roundworm)	Toxocariasis (visceral larva migrans)	dogs, cats	most mild & chronic; F, malaise, cough, bronchospasm (// Loeffler's), HSM, LN, endophthalmitis	orgs in granuloma Bx; serology	worldwide; esp pedes	albendazole
Trichinella	Trichinellosis	pigs	F, myalgia, rash, periorb edema (// <u>flu + facial edema</u>); dry cough, myocarditis	orgs in muscle Bx (classic spiral)	P-10,000,000	albendazole
Cestodes						
Diphyllobothrium (fish tapeworm)	Diphyllobothriasis	humans, bears, foxes [cyclops → fish] ∴ food-borne	most s Sx; D, megaloblastic anemia		P-10,000,000 Alaska, Canada	praziquantel
Echinococcus granulosus (dog tapeworm)	Echinococcosis (cystic or unilocular E, hydatid disease)	dogs [herbivores—sheep, cattle, pigs]	most s Sx until enlarge; S/Sx referable to liver (70%), lung (20%), other organs (10%)	US, CT; serology	P-2,700,000 including *E. multilocularis* grazing countries where dogs eat viscera	2–5% albendazole + praziquantel excision p CT
Echinococcus multilocularis	Echinococcosis (alveolar or multilocular E, hydatid disease)	foxes, dogs, cats [rodents]	most s Sx until enlarge; S/Sx referable to liver, lung, brain; local invasion // tumor → death	US, CT; serology	P-as above N hemis—FSU, central Eur, N Japan, Alaska	s Tx 90% c Tx 20% surgery
Hymenolepsis	Hymenolepiasis (dwarf tapeworm)	rodents [none]	most s Sx; abd pain, D	ova in stool	P-75,000,000 worldwide cities #1 human tapeworm in NA, LA	praziquantel
Taenia saginata	Taeniasis (beef tapeworm)	[cattle]	most s Sx	proglottid or ova in stool	P-77,000,000	praziquantel
Taenia solium	Taeniasis (pork tapeworm, cysticercosis)	[pigs]	adult worm (from eating pig cysticerci)—anorexia, abd pain; larvae (from FO transmission of ova)—S/Sx referable to muscle, brain (epilepsy, HA, psyc), other organs	proglottid or ova in stool; larvae in imaging & Bx; serology	P-10,000,000	praziquantel

		Trematodes					
fish [freshwater snails → fish] ∴ foodborne	*Clonorchis* or *Opisthorchis* (oriental liver fluke)	Clonorchiasis (Chinese liver fluke disease)	anorexia, biliary colic, HM, cirrhosis, ascites, jaundice, cholangitis, CA	ova in stool; serology	P-7,000,000 Asia		praziquantel
sheep, cattle [freshwater snails → plants] ∴ foodborne	*Fasciola hepatica* (liver fluke)	Fascioliasis	F, malaise, RUQ pain, biliary colic, HM, wt loss, jaundice, urticaria	ova in stool; serology	P-2,000,000 worldwide	10,000	triclabendazole
pigs [freshwater snails → plants] ∴ foodborne	*Fasciolopsis* (intestinal fluke)	Fasciolopsiasis	anorexia, DNV	ova in stool	P-15,000,000 SE Asia		praziquantel
dogs, cats, pigs [freshwater snails → crabs] ∴ foodborne	*Paragonimus* (lung fluke)	Paragonimiasis	malaise, urticarial rash → chronic cough, hemoptysis, pleuritic chest pain	ova in sputum or stool	P-20,000,000 worldwide foci China, Korea		praziquantel
humans (*S.m, S.h*); humans, dogs, cats, pigs, cattle, water buffalo, horses (*S.j*) [freshwater snails] ∴ percutaneous infection	*Schistosoma mansoni* (*S.m*), *hematobium* (*S.h*), *japonicum* (*S.j*), *et al* (*S.j*, blood fluke)	Schistosomiasis (bilharziasis, snail fever, Katayama fever)	F, urticaria, species specific Sx— terminal hematuria, obstructive uropathy (*S.h*); HSM, portal HTN, dysentery (*S.m*); Katayama F c̄ urticaria, D, HSM, cough (4 wks p̄ primary infection) (*S.j*)	ova in stool (*S.m, S.j*), midday terminal urine (*S.h*); serology	P-200,000,000 Africa, SE Asia, SA 85% in SSA *S.h > S.m > S.j > S.i > S.mek*	200,000	praziquantel

Invasive Ectoparasites

domestic, field hosts e.g. dogs, rats, humans (accidental) via direct contact with larva from eggs laid in soil or damp cloth	*Cordylobia* (tumbu fly, mango fly)	Myiasis	boils	none	SSA	topical petroleum jelly, forceps extraction
via direct contact with fly eggs from vector or intermediate vector (e.g. housefly)	*Dermatobia* (bot fly)	Myiasis	boils	none	LA	excision
via direct contact with adult mite	*Sarcoptes* (mite)	Scabies	papules, burrows	orgs on Px, micro	worldwide	permethrin
domestic, field hosts via direct contact with adult flea	*Tunga* (jigger flea, sand flea)	Myiasis (tungiasis)	pustules on toe webs	none	worldwide tropics	needle extraction

Protozoa

	Organism	Disease	Symptoms	Diagnosis	Epidemiology	US cases	Treatment
Enteric							
	Balantidium	Balantidiasis	D (dysentery) NV, cramps, tenesmus	trophs or cysts in wet or stained [stool]			metronidazole + iodoquinol
	Cryptosporidium parvum **BW (B)**	Cryptosporidiosis	chronic watery D esp in ICP	oocysts in AF stained [stool]		50,000	none
	Cyclospora cayatanesis **BW (B)**	Cyclosporosis	chronic watery D in ICP	oocysts in AF stained [stool]			TMP/SMZ
	Entamoeba histolytica **BW (B)**	Amoebiasis	most s Sx as ACPs; dysentery; liver abscess (gen s prior GI Sx, M > F)	trophs or cysts in wet or stained [stool]; serology	I-50,000,000 P-500,000,000 tropics c poor sanitation	70,000	metronidazole + iodoquinol
	Giardia lamblia **BW (B)**	Giardiasis	chronic watery D	cysts or trophs in stained [stool]; string test	I-500,000,000		metronidazole
	Isospora	Isosporosis	chronic watery D in ICP	cysts in AF stained [stool]			TMP/SMZ
Non-Enteric							
cats [sheep, goats, pigs, rodents, chickens]	*Toxoplasma gondii* **BW (B)**	Toxoplasmosis	most s Sx; mono-like—F, LN; congenital triad of hydrocephalus, cerebral calcification, chorioretinitis; encephalitis & chorioretinitis in OD	serology; PCR; orgs in tissue Bx	I-100,000,000 worldwide	300,000	pyrimethamine + sulfadiazine
	Trichomonas	Trichomoniasis	mucosal discharge	orgs in wet prep	I-175,000,000	0	metronidazole

Viruses

Disease	Agent	Transmission	Signs/Symptoms	Diagnosis	Epidemiology	Prevention/Notes
Hepatitis A	Hepatitis A virus (HAV) **BW (B)**	via FO	F, malaise, anorexia, NV, RUQ pain, jaundice; no chronic infection	serology	I-1,400,000	0.1–0.3% vaccine IG for PEP
Hepatitis B	hepatitis B virus (HBV)	via sexual, perinatal, IDU, nosocomial	F, malaise, anorexia, NV, RUQ pain, jaundice → acute fulminant (0.1–0.6%) c CFR 70%, chronic carriers (10%) → cirrhosis, HCC, hepatic failure	serology	I-5,000,000 P-250,000,000 chronic carriers 2 billion infected worldwide 75% in Asia	<1% 600,000 from Ca & cirrhosis vaccine HBIG for PEP
Hepatitis C	Hepatitis C virus (HCV)	via sexual, perinatal, IDU, nosocomial	Most s Sx → chronic carriers (80%) → cirrhosis, HCC, hepatic failure (// HBV)	serology	P-200,000,000 80% chronic carriers most in Asia	50,000 DAA no vaccine IG ineffective for PEP
Hepatitis D	Hepatitis D virus (HDV)	via sexual, perinatal, IDU, nosocomial	F, malaise, anorexia, NV, RUQ pain, jaundice → chronic carriers → cirrhosis, HCC, hepatic failure	serology	P-10,000,000	2–20% no vaccine IG, HBIG ineffective for PEP
Hepatitis E	hepatitis E virus (HEV)	via FO, esp from contaminated water	F, malaise, anorexia, NV, RUQ pain, jaundice; no chronic infections (// HAV)	serology	I-20,000,000 3,000,000 acute cases epidemic AR 7%	57,000 < 1% unless pregnant, then 20% in 3rd tri no vaccine IG ineffective for PEP
HIV/AIDS	human immuno-deficiency virus (HIV)	via sexual, perinatal, IDU, nosocomial	acute seroconversion over 1–2 wks c mac-pap rash (includes palms, soles), multiple Sx // mononucleosis; 4 stages—PGL → mild c mucocut Δs or HZ → intermediate c F, weight loss, chronic D → severe c AIDS, OIs	serology	I-1,900,000 P-35,000,000 70% in SSA (5% of all adults in the region)	1,500,000 from TB, OD 70% in SSA ART trial vaccine
Influenza	influenza virus (types A, B, C; only A subtypes cause pandemic)	via droplet nuclei	F, HA, myalgia, malaise, nonproductive cough, sore throat, rhinitis	virus isolation, IFA, RT-PCR, serology	I-5–10% non-pandemic	1,500,000 non-pandemic highest CFR U1 vaccine

via droplet nuclei	Morbillivirus	Measles	cough, coryza, conjunctivitis, Koplik's spots, rash d3 x 4 d; CP of D, pneumonia, croup, deafness, brain damage	serology	unknown SSA cool, rainy season except Sahel where peaks in dry season	100,000 0.1-5% in DCs; 10-30% in CEs with SAM vaccine
via FO	Poliovirus (types 1, 2, 3; type 2 eliminated in wild in 1999)	Poliomyelitis (infantile paralysis)	most s Sx (90–95%); F, HA, NV (4–8%); CP (< 1%) of myalgia, backache, asymmetric AFP LE > UE (0.1–0.5% c paralytic polio)	virus isolation from stool; serology	1-< 100 endemic in Pakistan, Afghanistan	5–10% c paralytic polio polyvalent vaccine

NB Disease incidence and prevalence estimates of chronic viruses and helminthes include subclinical infections for which asymptomatic carriers are common. For those infections, $P_{infection} > P_{disease}$

Reference

1. Yung, A. (2005). Golden rules of infectious diseases. In: A. Yung, M. McDonald, D. Spelman, et al. (Eds.), *Infectious diseases—a clinical approach*, 2nd ed. Hawthorn East, Victoria, Australia: IP Communications.

Annex 8.5
EPIDEMIC PREPAREDNESS AND RESPONSE

I. EPIDEMIC PREPAREDNESS

A. Prior to Seasonal Epidemic

1. Establish a National Coordinating Committee (NCC).
2. Designate a lead agency and lead official in the NCC.
3. Establish a Local Coordinating Committee (LCC).
4. Designate a lead official in the LCC.
5. Anticipate roles for partner agencies (e.g. inter-agency and team coordination, disease surveillance, field epidemiological investigation, laboratory identification, case management guideline development, outbreak logistics, public information, and social mobilization).
6. Identify sources of funds.
7. Intensify disease surveillance.
8. Identify reference lab(s) for communicable diseases of epidemic potential.
9. Ensure mechanism for specimen transport.

II. OUTBREAK RESPONSE

A. Initial Response to Suspected Outbreak

1. Form an emergency team to investigate and manage the outbreak
   a. identify key roles on the outbreak investigation team(s)
      (1) epidemiology and surveillance
      (2) case management
      (3) water and sanitation
      (4) laboratory services
      (5) communication
   b. staff those roles
      (1) epidemiologist—to monitor proper data collection and surveillance procedures
      (2) physician—to confirm clinical S/Sx and train health workers in case management
      (3) water and sanitation expert—to develop a plan for reducing sources of contamination
      (4) microbiologist—to take environmental/biological samples for laboratory confirmation, train health workers in proper sampling techniques, and confirm use of appropriate methods in the diagnostic laboratory
      (5) behavior change communication (BCC) specialist—to assess the population's reaction to the outbreak, create, and disseminate appropriate health messages

B. Outbreak Investigation Protocol

1. Establish access, contacts, logistics.
2. Verify outbreak.
3. Confirm diagnosis.
4. Develop case definition.
   a. What are most patients complaining of?
   b. Describe a typical patient.
   c. Choose a case definition from the community descriptions confirmed by your own observations.
5. Count cases and determine demographic data.
   a. How many people live in the outbreak area?
   b. Who are the patients?
   c. What is their background—age, sex?
   d. Where are the patients coming from?
   e. When did the patients arrive?

      f.   Why are the patients arriving?

      g.   Count the number of patients fitting the case definition.

      h.   Count the number of fresh graves or bodies at health facilities and inquire as to cause.

6.   Orient the descriptive data—person, place, and time.

      a.   Tabulate data on affected patients.

      b.   Make a spot map.

          (1)   When and where was/were the first reported case(s) seen indicating an outbreak?

      c.   Plot an epidemic curve.

          (1)   What is the present # of patients/day or week?

          (2)   What is the usual # of patients/day or week?

          (3)   Is this an increase?

          (4)   What is the present # of deaths/week or month?

          (5)   What is the usual # of deaths/week or month?

          (6)   Is this an increase?

      d.   Calculate attack rates and case fatality ratios for total patients, U5, O5, and gender.

7.   Develop hypothesis.

      a.   Postulate sources of disease and mechanism of spread.

      b.   Estimate the population at risk of contracting disease and of dying from it.
Consider especially:

          (1)   poor

          (2)   those with limited access to health services

          (3)   minorities

          (4)   malnourished

          (5)   pregnant and lactating

          (6)   infants not breast fed, children unvaccinated

          (7)   elderly

8.   Initiate control measures considering agent, host, and environment.

      a.   What action has the community taken?

      b.   Identify local response capacity.

          (1)   What number and type of staff are locally available?

          (2)   What drugs and supplies are locally available?

      c.   Determine immediate unmet needs.

          (1)   specimen collection and lab diagnosis

          (2)   logistics

          (3)   support for clinical care—staff, drugs, and supplies

          (4)   support for environmental health

      d.   Undertake further necessary actions.

          (1)   case management with secondary prevention

          (2)   patient isolation

          (3)   health education

          (4)   agent and reservoir identification

          (5)   environmental decontamination

          (6)   primary prevention

          (7)   public information

9.   Inform authorities with investigation report.

10.   Initiate ongoing disease surveillance.

C.   During Epidemic

1.   NCC should meet at least weekly.

2.   LCC should meet daily at first, then reduce meeting frequency as circumstances warrant.

D.   **Surveillance Systems Lessons Learned**

    1.   Start small, keep it simple

        a.   active surveillance at sentinel sites

        b.   simple standard operating procedures

            (1)   case investigation

            (2)   specimen collection

    2.   Invest in local people and systems

    3.   Focus the system on performance-based indicators

        a.   polio—non-polio acute flaccid paralysis detection rate of 1:100,000

        b.   gastroenteritis—stool specimen collection rate of 80%

    4.   Link data to action

        a.   case detection → local response

        b.   case locations → need for (sub)national immunization days

        c.   lab info → recognition of imported vs indigenous cases

        d.   other process indicators → system improvement

    5.   Show success, then expand

Annex 8.6
COMMUNICABLE DISEASE CONTROL

Glossary

ABX	antibiotics
AM	morning
AR	attack rate
ARI	acute respiratory infection
bd	twice daily
C&S	culture and antibiotic sensitivity
CFR	case fatality rate
CHW	community health worker
COTS	Cholera Outbreak Training and Shigellosis Program (training program developed at ICDDR)
CT	cholera toxin
d	day
D	diarrhea
DF	dengue fever
DOC	drug of choice
Dx	diagnosis
EHEC	enterohemorrhagic *E. coli*
EPI	Expanded Programme on Immunization
ETEC	enterotoxigenic *E. coli*
F	fever
h	hour
HPI	history of present illness
HUS	hemolytic-uremic syndrome
ICDDR	International Centre for Diarrhoeal Disease Research, Bangladesh
ID_{50}	median infective dose
IPD	inpatient department
IPT	intermittent preventive treatment
IRS	indoor residual spraying
ITN	insecticide treated net
IV	intravenous
IVF	intravenous fluids
L	liter
LCC	Local Coordinating Committee
MOH	Ministry of Health
N	nausea
N/A	not available
NCC	National Coordinating Committee
NGT	nasogastric tube
O5	over 5 year-old
OCV	oral cholera vaccine
OPD	outpatient department
ORS	oral rehydration salts/solution
p	person
PO	by mouth
PPE	personal protective equipment
PRN	as needed
Pt(s)	patient(s)
P_T	population total

q	every
qd	daily
rBS	recombinant beta subunit (of cholera toxin)
RDT	rapid diagnostic test
SD1	*S. dysenteriae* type 1
SSU	short stay unit
S/Sx	signs and symptoms
STEC	Shiga toxin producing *E. coli*
Sx	symptoms
T	temperature
U2	under 2 year-old
U5	under 5 year-old
V	vomiting
WHO	World Health Organization
YF	yellow fever
yr	year
Zn	zinc

DIARRHEA

Pathogens

Cholera

V. cholerae has > 200 serogroups. Serogroups are classified by biotype, and for serogroup O1, by serotype and biotype. Humans are the only known vertebrate host for cholera, and only serogroups O1 and O139 cause epidemic disease. There is no clinical difference between them. Other serogroups may cause disease in individuals, but not epidemics. When a suspected cholera serotype (strain) is isolated in the lab, one of the first tests performed is bacterial agglutination with O1 and O139 antisera. Strains are thereby identified as *V. cholerae* O1, O139, or non-O1/non-O139.

- If (+) agglutination to O1 antisera, then the strain is further tested for agglutination to antiserum of Ogawa and Inaba serotypes.
- If (+) agglutination to O139 antisera, then the strain is not further subdivided (except as producer or non-producer of CT as noted below).
- If (−) agglutination to O1 and O139 antisera, then the strain is known as non-O1, non-O139 *V. cholerae*.

A strain is further identified as a producer or non-producer of cholera toxin (CT). CT production is a major determinant of disease development. Strains lacking CT do not produce epidemics even if from the O1 or O139 serogroup.

- Serogroup O1 exists as 2 main biotypes—classical and El Tor—though hybrids also exist. Each biotype occurs as two serotypes—Ogawa and Inaba. Classic biotype caused the 5th and 6th pandemics but little epidemic disease since the 1970s though it still causes cases in India. **El Tor biotype** caused the 7th (current) pandemic and almost all recent outbreaks. El Tor was first isolated in 1905 in El Tor, Egypt after importation by Indonesian pilgrims travelling to Mecca. It survives longer in the environment and produces CT similar to the classical biotype. Presumably because of CT pathogenicity, the % of cholera patients with severe disease has doubled over the past 10 yrs. These patients tend to require IV fluid therapy.
- Serogroup O139 may have evolved from strains of O1 El Tor as they share many properties though not agglutination. In spring of 2002 in Dhaka, O139 cases exceeded O1 El Tor cases for the first time, and it was postulated that O139 may become the cause of an 8th pandemic. However, since then, O1 has again become dominant.

Infective dose depends on individual susceptibility. Relevant host factors include immunity produced by prior infection with serogroup O1 as well as stomach acidity. ID_{50} may be 100,000 orgs, so personal hygiene plays a lesser role than in shigellosis where the ID_{50} is much lower.

Shigella

Shigella has 4 species.

- *S. dysenteriae* type 1 (SD1 or Shiga bacillus) causes the severest disease of all *Shigella* sp because of its neurotoxin (Shiga toxin), longer duration of illness, higher ABX resistance, higher CFR thru invasive complications, and great epidemic potential.
- *S. flexneri* is the most common, and is generally endemic, in developing countries
- *S. sonnei* is the most common in industrial countries
- *S. boydii* and *S. sonnei* give mild disease.

Table 8.6.1
Shigella Species

Species	Serogroup	Serotypes	Notes
S. dysenteriae	A	1–15	SD1 gives most severe disease with complications of HUS
S. flexneri	B	1–6 (15 subtypes)	Greatest burden of disease and main cause of endemic shigellosis
S. boydii	C	1–18	Mild disease
S. sonnei	D	1	Mild disease

ID_{50} may be 10 orgs, so personal hygiene plays a greater role than in cholera.

E. coli

Some kinds of *E. coli* produce a Shiga toxin. Shiga toxin genes reside in bacteriophage genome integrated into the bacterial chromosome. Some ABX, e.g. fluoroquinolones, induce expression of phage genes. The bacteria that make these toxins are variously called "Shiga toxin-producing *E. coli*" (STEC), "enterohemorrhagic *E. coli*" (EHEC), or "vero-cytotoxic *E. coli*" (VTEC). All terms refer to the same group of bacteria.

*   *E. coli* O157:H7 (often called "*E. coli* O157" or "O157") is the most commonly identified STEC in North America, and it causes most *E. coli* outbreaks. Approximately 5–10% of EHEC infections result in HUS.
*   Non-O157 STEC serogroups also cause disease. In the USA, serogroups O26, O111, and O103 are the most commonly identified *E. coli* pathogens overall.

Epidemiology

Diarrhea epidemiology is seasonally dependent. Environmental temperature directly influences biologic activity—$\Delta 5°C$ is proportional to 3× risk of disease

*   temperate climates: bacterial diarrhea in warmer, humid season; rotavirus diarrhea in cooler, dry season
*   tropical climates: bacterial diarrhea in rainy season; rotavirus diarrhea year round with increased incidence in cooler season
*   most common pathogens for watery diarrhea—rotavirus, ETEC, *V. cholerae*; most important pathogen for epidemic watery diarrhea—*V. cholerae*
*   most common pathogens for dysentery—shigella species, salmonella species, *Campylobacter jejuni*, *Clostridium difficile*, EIEC, EHEC, *E. coli* O157:H7, *Entamoeba histolytica*, *Yersinia enterocolitica*; most important pathogens for epidemic dysentery—*S. dysenteriae* serotype 1 (developing countries), *E. coli* O157:H7 (developed countries)

Bangladesh has two seasonal cholera peaks: pre-monsoon with hot, humid weather (esp weeks 15–20 in Apr-May) creating increased biological activity; post-monsoon (esp weeks 30–40 in Aug–Sep) with contamination of water sources. Pre-monsoon epidemics are generally worse than post-monsoon ones. Dysentery has low level year-round incidence, but epidemics occur roughly each decade. Epidemic strains display new, additive antibiotic resistance which probably triggers the epidemic. Once resistant strains have become endemic, antibiotic susceptibility rarely reappears. SD1 acquires resistance quickly. *Sf* acquires it more slowly, and that resistance may wane with decreasing ABX pressure.

At ICDDR, annual proportional incidence approximates the following:

Table 8.6.2
Proportional Incidence of Diarrheal Pathogens in Bangladesh

Total		Pedes	
Rotavirus	30%	Rotavirus	45%
Cholera (O1 >> O139)	20%	*E. coli*	45%
ETEC	15%	Camplyobacter	10%
Shigella (flexneri >> boydii, sonnei, SD1)	5%		
Other	30%		

*   *E. coli* overall = 35% of cases, but ETEC = 15%.
*   *E. coli* tends to dominate before monsoon season and flooding.
*   Cholera tends to dominate after monsoon season and flooding.
*   Overall, 60–70% of diarrhea cases may be vaccine-preventable.
*   30% of Pts have no pathogen identified.

Preventive Medicine

Clean water and waste management for cholera.
Personal hygiene (hand washing with soap and clean towels) for shigella.

Water	safe drinking water (boiled, chlorinated)
	NB Sphere standards are not enough—you need increased quantities of chlorinated water at household level.
San	clean latrines for safe disposal of excreta
	hand washing with soap
Food	safe food (cooked, stored)
	breast feeding

Fomites safe disposal of dead bodies with disinfection of clothing

NB After outbreak of a fecal-oral pathogen, food hygiene and funereal practices may influence human-to-human transmission more then water quality.

Health education to affected population

Wash hands with soap:

after using toilets/latrines.

after disposing of children's feces.

before preparing food.

before eating.

before feeding children.

Boil or disinfect water with chlorine solution. (Bottle it, boil it, ferment it, or forget it.)

Eat only freshly cooked food. (Peel it, cook it, or leave it.)

Do not defecate near water sources.

Use latrines and keep them clean.

Consider vaccination for areas and populations most at risk. Pre-emptive vaccination for new arrivals (esp nutritionally impaired IDPs) moving into an endemic area is increasingly accepted. Reactive vaccination where cholera has broken out is more controversial—particularly if vaccine stocks are not locally available and remain limited worldwide. There are 2 types of oral cholera vaccines licensed internationally: one with dead *V. cholerae*, and one with live *V. cholerae*. (Parenteral cholera vaccine is not recommended because of low protective efficacy and frequent severe adverse reactions.)

Killed whole cell *V. cholerae* O1 vaccine

- Dukoral—mixture of the classical biotype (both Inaba and Ogawa serotypes) and the El Tor biotype (only Inaba serotype) + purified recombinant B-subunit of CT (rBS)

  Dose: 3 cc vaccine given in 150 cc of buffer solution; 2 doses, 1–6 wks apart; cold chain required. The regime is identical for all patients, and thus can't be given to pedes < 2 yr because of volume loading.

  Dukoral has been the main vaccine considered for use in high-risk populations.

- mORC-VAX and Shanchol—similar to Dukoral except they do not contain the rBS, hence do not require a buffer, and are 1/3 the cost to produce. mORC-VAX, produced in Vietnam, is derived from a vaccine administered to millions of people since 1997, but is not WHO pre-qualified, and is not expected to have international distribution. Shanchol, produced in India, has international distribution (e.g. used in the Haiti cholera vaccination campaign of 2012), and is now the agent of choice for WHO. It confers immunity 10d p 2nd dose, effectiveness > 85% at 6 mo, and protection > 50% at 5 yr. Also confers short-term protection vs ETEC. Dose: 1.5 cc vaccine followed by water ingestion but no fasting needed; 2 doses, 2 wks apart; cold chain required except for day of use.

Live-attenuated genetically modified *V. cholerae* O1 vaccine

- Orochol—bivalent formulation as in Dukoral without rBS of CT.

  Dose: single dose. No longer manufactured.

WHO recommendations: "Vaccination should not disrupt the provision of other high-priority health interventions to control or prevent cholera outbreaks. Vaccines provide a short-term effect that can be implemented to bring about an immediate response while the longer term interventions of improving water and sanitation, which involve large investments, are put into place" [1].

ICDDR recommendations: "Because of limitations in terms of transport, formulation, and cost of the current Dukoral vaccine, the COTS program does NOT require the utilization of the vaccine during an outbreak; it is NOT necessary to vaccinate to overcome an outbreak. However, if Dukoral is readily available and staff are properly trained in its use according to the guidelines that come with the vaccine, the COTS program PERMITS Dukoral's use (ideally before an outbreak) in the following high-risk populations: refugee populations in which cholera is present, health care workers managing cholera cases, and communities in which the incidence rate is greater than 1 in 1000 annually" [2].

Epidemiological Surveillance

Cholera

Epidemiological assumptions (WHO, COTS):

Estimated attack rates
    10–20% extremely vulnerable hosts and poor environmental health (WHO)
    5% (refugee camps with malnutrition) (COTS)
    2% (rural communities of < 5000 p) (COTS)
    1% (severe epidemic—good estimate of ultimate disease burden) (WHO)
    0.6% (endemic areas with bad sanitation) (COTS)
    0.2% (endemic areas in open settings—suitable for initial calculations of early resource requirements)
    NB   Overall, 90% of cases are mild and difficult to distinguish from other types of D.
    NB   Asymptomatic carriers are very common (10x # of cases).

Referral rates for IVs   20% of cases (much higher—70% at ICDDR as it shortens recovery time)

Case fatality ratios   1% (with good care)

The following catchment populations will yield 100 acute Pts of whom 20 will be severely dehydrated:
    refugee camp of 2000 people (AR of 5% = 100 Pts)
    open settings in endemic area with 50,000 people (AR 0.2% = 100 Pts)

A population of 100,000 infected individuals in an epidemic area will yield the following (WHO):

Population infected	100,000
Clinical cases	1,000 + (1% of infected population)
Cases needing early resources	200 + (20% of cases)
Cases needing IV therapy	200 + (20% of cases, 0.2% of infected population)
Anticipated deaths	10 + (1% CFR)

NB   In non-endemic areas, AR adults > AR pedes because adults have higher exposure risks.
    In endemic areas, AR pedes > AR adults because adults have been exposed since childhood.

Clinical Medicine

Delivery of Health Services

Active case finding through CHWs
Treatment facilities—2 types
    outpatient ORS center
        ORS packets, Zn
        clean water
        ABX (in the case of a shigellosis outbreak)
        recording form for demographic information
        trained staff (nurse, health aides)
        if budget allows:
            soap to give to families (especially in the case of a shigellosis outbreak)
            communication (radio, telephone) with the treatment facility for patients who need transfer, and means of transport (ambulance, horse, rickshaw, etc.)
    inpatient treatment facility (section of existing hospital/health center or makeshift facility)
        one way traffic flow—from triage to OPD/home and IPD
        running water or close proximity to water source
        large quantities of safe water (40–60 L/p/d)
        adequate waste disposal system
        shelter from weather
        recording form for patient demographic information and clinical status
        IVs, suspension lines, ORS, meds, and other essential supplies in treatment areas

trained staff (physicians, nurses, health aides, and cleaners) with supervision of Pts 24/7

fee waiver policy for emergencies

1 family carer or visitor/Pt

Standardized Case Management

Suspected cholera outbreak definition

   Pt > 5 yr develops acute watery diarrhea with severe dehydration or death,

   any sudden increase in the daily # of patients with acute watery diarrhea especially if they pass typical rice-water stools

Case definitions

   cholera where the disease is not known to be present

      Pt > 5 yr with acute watery diarrhea plus severe dehydration or death

   cholera where the disease is confirmed present

      Pt > 2 yr with acute watery diarrhea

   bacillary dysentery

      Pt with acute diarrhea plus visible blood in the stool

Treatment protocols

   Overview

         assess for dehydration

         rehydrate the Pt

         maintain hydration by replacing ongoing fluid losses until diarrhea stops

         give an oral antibiotic to the Pt with severe dehydration

         feed the Pt

   Triage by dehydration status

         1/3 Pts without dehydration → OPD for ORS

         2/3 Pts with dehydration   → SSU for IVF, ORS

                                       → IPD for adults with D > 14d, typhoid fever, meningitis;

                                             pedes with malnutrition + infectious complications

   HPI & stool appearance help make presumptive Dx

      Shigella HPI: 3 d of Sx with F + abdominal pain/cramps + bloody D (not voluminous) + tenesmus (from colonic mucosal inflammation and erosions), anorexia ± dehydration.

         Stools: chunky style with visible coagulated blood (related to coagulation necrosis in bowel). However, watery diarrhea may appear early in the illness.

      Cholera HPI: 6 h of Sx onset in early morning with V, profuse watery D without pain or cramps, marked dehydration.

         Stools: homogeneous rice water, occasionally turbid with fine particulate, occasionally yellow-ish when mixed with urine.

      Vibrio parahemolyticus

         Stools: "meat-washed stool" treated similar to cholera

      Rotavirus

         HPI: V without F

         Stools: look like mashed pulses

      Amoeba Stools: appears dark brown because the parasite oxidizes heme.

   IVF   ASAP (< 1 min) if severely dehydrated. 75+% of Pts with dehydration at ICDDR get IVs because they feel better more quickly. Otherwise PO sufficient. NGT OK if IV and PO are unsuccessful (very rare).

   NB   acetate in cholera saline may cause hypocalcemia and tetany.

   ORS for rehydration

         Pt < 6 months, glucose ORS

         Pt > 6 months, rice-based ORS

   Zn   Pt < 6 months, 10 mg PO qd × 10–14 d

         Pt > 6 months to 5 yr, 20 mg PO qd × 10–14 d

ABX   always given under physician supervision
      Cholera
      In epidemic season, use ABX × 1 dose with all dehydrated patients with suspected cholera.
      In non-epidemic season, use clinical judgment on watery diarrhea.
      If organism is sensitive, doxycycline is generally DOC. ICDDR has used azithro as DOC in all ages.
      Dysentery
      Use ABX for dysentery year round (if resources limited, prioritize high risk groups—U5, malnourished, toxic, post-measles, pregnant, old, etc.). If organism is sensitive, cipro is generally DOC. ICDDR has used cipro in adults and pivmecillinam in pedes. Ceftriaxone is 2nd choice for both age groups.
      Rotavirus
      Usually, no ABX, unless Pt is very ill and clinical picture suggests combined disease.
      ETEC
      Usually, no ABX, unless Pt develops severe dehydration.

Misc Sx V   no antiemetics, but use NGT or IVF if Pt ultimately can't take PO
        F   ± antipyretics depending upon resources available
      Physician rounds q 2 h on severely ill Pts; 4×/d on Pts with some dehydration (SSU); 2×/d on Pts without dehydration (OPD).

Disposition
      Cholera improves quickly—young Pts get off IVF by 24 h, old Pts by 48 h.
      ETEC lasts for 3–5 d.
      Shigella dysentery lasts for 3–5 d if uncomplicated.
      Rotavirus lasts for 5 d until kids can feed again (strips off brush border). Maternal motivation is important during this time.
      Overall, rice-based ORS ends up adequately treating 85% of diarrheas

Discharge
      no dehydration, < purging, able to take ORS adequately
      5–7% return visits are expected; > 10% return visits mean discharge policy is too aggressive

Essential drugs & supplies
      cholera kits
      drug choices driven by culture data (10–20 specs)

Referral guidelines
      refer all Pts refractory to rehydration and standard ABX to hospital for C&S

Secondary prevention for the discharged patient
      ORS liberally distributed with instructions for use—2 ORS sachets to all discharged Pts (home based salt solution is dangerous)
      soap distribution to accompanying persons

Secondary prevention at the site
      Isolate the affected Pt/ward/camp/defecation area.
      Impose hand washing upon entry/exit to affected hut/clinic/camp/defecation area, etc. (0.05% Cl).
            In-service staff—HCWs should not handle food or water (ORS); kitchen staff should not handle hospital waste.
      Recruit cleaners, establish cleaning routine (0.5% Cl).
            wash spills ASAP
            wash floor q 4 h
            collect stool collection buckets bd or PRN (wash them with 2.0% Cl)
            change and wash cot covers qd
            wash cots after each Pt
            spray the affected area qd (water storage containers, water distribution points, latrines, door handles, etc. in clinic, camp, and defecation area)
      Identify body fluid disposal site (2.0% Cl).
            hold Cl treated fluids 2 h before dumping
      Establish hygienic funereal practices (2.0% Cl).

Epidemic Management

Outbreak investigation protocol in place
    rapid response teams to investigate case reports
    epidemic investigation kits to mobilize
    specimens to collect
    labs to confirm Dx of *V. cholerae*, *S. dysenteriae*, other shigella, and *E. coli* O157:H7
        dipstick identification on representative sample of specs is useful for cholera, but C&S is essential because dipsticks are not available for shigella, ETEC. Vibrio are hardy if kept moist and cool. They can survive a week in Cary Blair media. Shigella are fragile and difficult to recover if transport time > 1 d.
        5–10 isolates initially to confirm outbreak
        30–50 isolates initially to create ABX use policy (bacterial resistance renders cotrimoxazole, amp/amox, nalidixic acid, and tetracycline unusable)
        20–30 isolates monthly from IPD and OPD before ABX therapy to assess evolving ABX resistance
        10–20 isolates periodically to reference laboratory to confirm ABX resistance patterns and undertake molecular studies
        20 isolates at end of the outbreak to confirm that new diarrheas are not epidemic pathogens
        NB   Systematic sampling is most representative—e.g. every 10th Pt or all Pts q 2 weeks adjusted as needed to collect the necessary specs.
            Sensitivity >> important than specificity in RDT screening during an epidemic.
            Pts from one geographic area are more likely to constitute a cluster involving a new pathogen.
            An area may be considered cholera-free after 2 incubation periods (total of 10 d) have passed without cholera disease. However, hospital monitoring should continue for a year due to tendency of enteric pathogens to re-emerge long after they are declared gone.
            Cholera may be viable but nonculturable from the environment; environmental monitoring has many false negatives.
        consider improvements to existing diagnostic labs
    hotlines set up for reporting of rumor
Health reference and educational materials in place
    case definitions
    case management and referral guidelines for communicable diseases with epidemic potential
    Pt, provider, and community educational materials
    specimen handling protocols
Epidemic command & control center established under local health authorities using principles and practices of incident mgmt
    unified command of multi-disciplinary specialists
    information channel to government and stakeholders
    support by government for technical actions
Coordination with technical sectors—particularly WASH (CFR is a function of case mgmt, but AR overall is a function of WASH)
    water supply, purification, and distribution systems
    bucket chlorination is low tech but reasonable way to reach individual HH or small communities
    water treatment units need Ca hypochlorite, chlorimetric, and colimetric monitoring devices
    chlorinators worth considering at water sources of high public demand and epidemic activity
    hygiene promoters with environmental health assessors to address hand and food hygiene in communities around the outbreak area (think ring vaccination with knowledge)
    safe disposal of medical waste and infectious sludge from treatment facilities
Medical logistics–resource prepositioning and stockpiles
    cots (take one and have carpenter make copies)
    plastic sheets with defecation hole or sleeve
    buckets (white color for stool—enables recognition of diarrhea color; different color for emesis; different color for domestic waste)
    IVF, IV sets, IV poles or suspension cords (cholera kits)

ORS powder and ORS vats (> 50 L)

cups, spoons

NGTs, syringes

soap cleaning supplies

bleaching powder (e.g. Ca hypochlorite)—chlorinate water sources where feasible, otherwise bucket chlorinate at untreated sources

equipment (e.g. chlorimetric and colimetric monitors)

Information management

update local authorities

intensify disease surveillance (health authorities, WHO)

issue health advisories (health & political authorities)

establish cholera advisory task force

reinforce training of public health cadres on diarrhea prevention and control.

reinforce education of clinicians on diarrhea case management and secondary prevention

Initiate public awareness and health education campaign

message content—WHO Cholera manual or COTS card for Health Promotion Worker)

messages dissemination—printed, loudspeaker, broadcast, community groups

messages uptake—community understands hand washing, ORS use, and 2 prevention measures

OCV   Cholera epidemic brings huge political pressures to DO something. This often translates into a hastily conceived vaccination campaign that distracts from core principles of cholera management. For every symptomatic Pt, there are 90–99 asymptomatic carriers, and the affected community is already extensively infected. Cholera vaccination, under these circumstances, has little public health benefit for the resource investment. If undertaken, the following will apply:

Vaccination campaign requires numerous staff. Community mobilizers are key. Clinical staff should not be poached from their clinical duties. Supervisors must be free to move at will.

Logistics is key—if the 1st day goes bad, the campaign goes bad.

Mark the domiciles which are done.

Hold after-action meetings each day.

Last day, use mobilizers with mobile broadcasting to find those missed.

Second phase vaccination should include CHWs with multi-purpose messages on water and sanitation.

Key lessons in epidemic response

Avoid: press exaggeration

ABX prophylaxis

reliance on IVF and insufficient ORS

lab investigation of cases once epidemic etiology is ascertained

prolonged hospitalization

hospital discharge criteria requiring multiple negative stool cultures

enthusiasm for OCV during epidemic

exaggerated water purification objectives

concentration of technical competencies in MOH at expense of districts

failure to share information with district stakeholders

References

1. World Health Organization. (2010). Cholera vaccines: WHO position paper. *Weekly Epidemiological Record* 85(13), 117–128.
2. International Centre for Diarrhoeal Disease Research, Bangladesh, and Swiss Tropical Institute (Eds). Cholera outbreak training and shigellosis (COTS) program [CD-ROM version 1.0, undated]. Available from the International Centre for Diarrhoeal Disease Research, Bangladesh, and http://www.cotsprogram.com.

INFLUENZA

Pathogens

Influenza viruses comprise 3 genera—influenza types A, B, and C—each with 1 species.

- Influenza type A is divided into subtypes based upon serological response to hemagglutinin (HA) and neuraminidase (NA) glycoproteins. There are 16 different HA subtypes and 9 different NA subtypes. H1N1, H2N2, and H3N2 are responsible for the major human pandemics in the last century. H2N2 virus circulated between 1957 and 1968 but currently does not. Only influenza A subtypes infect birds, and all subtypes can do so. Bird flu viruses do not usually infect humans. But, in 1997, an outbreak of H5N1 avian influenza in poultry in Hong Kong marked the first known direct human transmission of avian influenza virus from birds to humans. Since then, H5, H7, and H9 avian influenza subtypes have been shown to infect humans.
- Influenza type B is morphologically similar to A and also creates seasonal and epidemic disease.
- Influenza type C is rare but can cause local epidemics.

Seasonal human influenza vaccine currently has 3 strains—H1N1/H3N2/B.

Influenza disease in humans has a short incubation period (1–3 d). Early symptoms are non-specific. It is highly infectious, especially early in the course of the disease, with a large # of asymptomatic carriers. Transmission potential (R_0) is a function of infectivity, period of contagiousness, daily contact rate, and host immunity. In general, the faster the transmission, the less feasible is interrupting transmission thru usual disease control tools of case finding, isolation, contact tracing, and ring vaccination.

Table 8.6.3
R_0 of Different Diseases (adapted from CDC [1])

Disease	R_0
Measles	12–18
Polio	5–7
Rubella	6–7
Diphtheria	6–7
Smallpox	5–7
Mumps	4–7
SARS	3 (excluding superspreaders)
Influenza pandemic	2–3 (1918)
Influenza seasonal	1.5–3

Table 8.6.4
Disease Comparison (adapted from US DHHS [2])

Attribute	Disease		
	Influenza	**Smallpox**	**SARS**
Transmissibility	Hi	Med	Low
R_0	> 2 (estimated 1.8 for 1918 pandemic)	5–7	3 (excluding superspreaders)
Geography	Widespread, multi-focal epidemics		Focal epidemics
Transmission location	Community		Within families and health care settings
Incubation period	1–3 days	10–12 days (CDC)	7–10 days
Attack rate	10–35%	58% (CDC)	Low
CFR	1% (seasonal) 50% (highly pathogenic avian influenza)	50% (unvaccinated) 30% (vaccinated post exposure) 11% (>20 y before exposure) 1.4 % (0–10 y before exposure)	5–10%
Epidemic investigation	Unlikely to track spread based upon movement of infected persons or contacts	High ability to track spread based upon movement of infected persons or contacts	Potential ability to track spread based upon movement of infected persons or contacts

Interventions to prevent transmission	International travel restrictions/screening possible but unlikely to prevent pandemic; quarantine unlikely; school closing and limits on public events likely; vaccination of priority groups	Vaccination effective if given within 4 d of infection	International travel restrictions/screening possible and likely to help prevent outbreaks; quarantine likely; school closing and limits on public events unlikely
Disruption of transportation infrastructure, community services	Widespread, widespread		Widespread, little

Preventive Medicine

Vaccination when available, social distancing, cough etiquette, hand hygiene

Epidemiological Surveillance

Rapid case investigation, contact tracing, and the containment of small clusters of cases
Quick reporting of suspected cases by affected countries

Clinical Medicine

Delivery of Health Services

Passive case finding but use of influenza clinics and fever hospitals

Standardized Case Management

Case definitions
Treatment protocols
    technical expertise in case management including rational use of antiviral treatment and prophylaxis
Essential drugs
    monitoring for counterfeit antiviral medications
Referral guidelines
    what to do in resource poor settings
Secondary prevention
    health care setting
        Pt isolation in specific hospital/ward designations
        private room or cohorting with other flu Pts
        minimize transport of Pt outside room
        limit # of HCWs interacting with flu Pt
        limit # of visitors interacting with flu Pt
        infection control
            standard   standard precautions with PPE and hand washing
            contact   hand hygiene
            airborne (droplet nuclei)   powered air purifying or N95 respirators, cough suppression
            droplet   N95 respirators
    home settings
        voluntary Pt isolation in private room
        minimize transport of Pt outside room
        limit # of family interacting with flu Pt
        infection control
            standard   standard precautions with PPE and hand washing
            contact   hand hygiene
            airborne (droplet nuclei)   N95 respirators, cough suppression
            droplet   N95 respirators
        voluntary quarantine of contacts of known cases

NB   management of contacts (contact tracing, contact monitoring) potentially useful only very early in epidemic

quarantine of close contacts for a complete incubation period potentially useful only very early in epidemic

all settings—try to decrease potential for infection

vaccination

seasonal or post-exposure antiviral chemoprophylaxis

< susceptibility to infection by 30%

if infection occurs, < infectiousness by 36%

if disease occurs, < probability of clinically recognizable Sx by 65%

Epidemic Management

Case definitions may change and become more specific as epidemic evolves

Case management guidelines for communicable diseases with epidemic potential

Outbreak management protocol

rapid response teams to investigate case reports

epidemic investigation kits to mobilize

specimens to collect

labs to verify diagnosis and share specimens with peer labs

Pts to identify, isolate, and treat (IPD and OPD settings)

contacts to trace and ? quarantine

hotline use and rumor investigation

Secondary prevention

specific groups of exposed or at risk in the community—most likely to work when there is limited disease transmission in the area, most cases can be traced to a specific contact or setting, and intervention is considered likely to slow the spread of disease

eg   quarantine of groups of people at known common source exposure (e.g. airplane, school, workplace, hospital, public gathering; ensure delivery of medical care, food, and social services to persons in quarantine with special attention to vulnerable groups) (useless once there is community-based spread)

eg   containment measures at specific sites or buildings of disease exposure (focused measures to > social distance)

cancel public events (concerts, sports, movies)

close buildings (recreational facilities, youth clubs)

restrict access to certain sites or buildings

community-wide measures (affecting exposed and non-exposed)—most likely to work where there is moderate to extensive disease transmission in the area, many cases cannot be traced, cases are increasing, and there is delay between Sx onset and case isolation.

eg   infection control measures

ARI etiquette—cover nose/mouth during cough or sneeze, use tissues, wash hands

avoidance of public gatherings by persons at high risk of complications

NB   use of masks by well persons is not recommended

eg   "snow" (stay-at-home) days and self-shielding (reverse quarantine) for initial 10 d period of community outbreak—may reduce transmission without explicit activity restrictions

eg   closure of schools, offices, large group gatherings, public transport (pedes more likely to transmit disease than adults)

NB   community quarantine (cordon sanitaire)—restriction of travel in and out of an area is unlikely to prevent introduction or spread of disease

international travel

NB   travel advisories to restrict international travel are generally useless in slowing epidemic spread

NB   health screening for fever and respiratory Sx at ports of entry is also generally useless in slowing epidemic spread

Resource prepositioning, stockpiles, and supply chain management
- facemasks
- PPE
- vaccines, antiviral drugs

Information management
- health workers
- political authorities
- public via awareness campaign and behavior change communication

Contingency planning
- incident/event management system and role designations
- surveillance, investigation, and containment
- vaccines, antivirals
- provision of essential services (lifelines, health care, and emergency response)
- culturally appropriate corpse management

Avian Influenza

Poultry epidemic
- Biosecurity
- Cull
- Disposal
- Disinfection
- Control movement
- Quarantine
- Count (surveillance around affected flocks)
- Ring vaccination

Overall
- primary prevention: animal vaccination (prevents viral reassortment)
  - cases: biosecurity (of premises), cull, disposal (of carcasses), disinfection (of premises)
  - contacts: quarantine, control movement, count (surveillance), ring vaccination

Human epidemic
- Health Care—infection control (PPE)
- Control movement
- Quarantine
- Count (surveillance)
- Vaccines
- Antiviral drugs

Overall
- primary prevention: animal vaccination (prevents viral reassortment)
- cases: isolation -> infection control, antiviral therapy
- contacts: quarantine, infection control, count (surveillance), vaccination, antivirals—chemoprophylaxis for high risk persons
- NB: travel screening & restrictions, quarantine, and school cancellation are not effective control measures.

References

1. World Health Organization and Centers for Disease Control and Prevention. History and epidemiology of global smallpox eradication. In: *Smallpox: Disease, prevention, and intervention training course*, undated. Retrieved from https://emergency.cdc.gov/agent/smallpox/training/overview/pdf/eradicationhistory.pdf
2. US Department of Health and Human Services. *Pandemic influenza preparedness and response plan draft*. Annex 12, p 8–11. August 2004. Retrieved from US Department of Health and Human Services, Washington, DC.

MALARIA

Pathogen Vectors

Table 8.6.5
Mosquito Biology [1]

Vector Group	Species	Breeding Sites	Resting Sites	Transmission Activity	Blood Source	Diseases
Anophelines	*Anopheles*	natural pools of unpolluted water	indoor/outdoor	evening and night	humans and animals	malaria, filariasis arboviruses
Culicines	*Aedes*	water containers (tires), pools of stagnant water	indoor/outdoor	day	humans and animals	filariasis, YF, DF
	Culex	organically polluted water (sewers), natural pools of unpolluted water	indoor/outdoor	day and night	humans and animals	filariasis, viral encephalitis
	Mansonia	unpolluted water with plants	indoor/outdoor	day and night	humans and animals	filariasis

Source: M Connolly (ed) in *Communicable disease control in emergencies—a field manual* © 2005. Used with permission of the World Health Organization.

Anopheles vector biology

egg becomes adult mosquito	9 d
adult mosquito becomes infective	12 d after bite on infected host
susceptible human host becomes infective	9 d after bite from infected mosquito
∴ earliest human clinical disease	30 d after eggs are laid

Preventive Medicine

Health messages
> Follow the 4-D rule:
>> **d**usk and **d**awn stay indoors as much as possible with window screens in good repair
>> **d**ress in light colored long sleeve shirts and long pants when outside
>> **D**EET (N,N-diethyl-M-toluamide) based mosquito repellants
>> **d**rain any standing water from the area (flower pots, old tires, clogged rain gutters, etc.); flush troughs, birdbaths, wading pools, etc. every 3 days

Insecticide
> 10% DDT, 1% malathion, 1% permethrin
> insecticide treated nets (ITNs) (esp long-lasting nets with duration of 3–5 years)
> indoor residual spraying (IRS) (esp within 2 weeks of high transmission season; more effective in Asia than Africa; not appropriate for dengue)

>> deterrence: # mosquitoes which don't enter room
>> repellence: # mosquitoes which enter then leave room
>> bite inhibition: # mosquitoes which enter room but don't bite
>> direct knock down: # mosquitoes which are knocked down, but still live
>> direct death: # mosquitoes killed

> NB   aerial spraying & outdoor spraying (fogging) are not especially useful in malaria
>> deterrence & repellence effectiveness is species-specific (e.g. aedes > anopheles > culex)
>> coils work by knockdown effect, not bite inhibition

Larvicide
> organophosphate (Temephos—safe for drinking water)
> *Bacillus thuringiensis israelensis* (bacterial toxin)
> *Mesocyclops* copepods (used in Vietnam in village water tanks)
> larvivorous fish (used in China in domestic water tanks)

Insect repellents (useful for individuals who can afford it but not as public health intervention)
    DEET
Chemoprophylaxis
    international staff travelling to endemic areas
    intermittent preventive treatment (IPT) for pregnant women in endemic areas where continuous chemoprophylaxis is
        not feasible
Generally, control programs rely upon:
    3 major components—ITN, IPT, and prompt clinical treatment
    2 ancillary components—IRS, environmental clean-up of breeding sites

Epidemiological Surveillance

Geographic reconnaissance
    mapping of target area before spraying
    mapping of homes for IRS
Entomological survey
    night mosquito survey
        # mosquitoes trapped/hr (calculation of man-biting rate)
        species identification
        mosquito dissection (F only) to determine parity; % parity inversely related to spraying effectiveness
Malariometric survey
    prevalence in sample of 100 persons
    spleen rate in sample of 100 persons
    slide positivity rate (ratio of # confirmed cases/# clinically suspected cases)
    proportion of fever caused by malaria (# fever cases with confirmed parasitemia/# total fevers)
Malaria mortality (# malaria deaths/10,000 p/d for given area)
Case fatality rate in all malaria cases
Case fatality rate in severe malaria cases
Proportional mortality (# malaria deaths/# total deaths)
Malaria incidence rate

Clinical Medicine

Delivery of Health Services

Active case finding through CHWs

Standardized Case Management

Case definition
    Pt with F or history of F associated with Sx such as N, V, D, headache, back pain, chills, myalgia, where other infec-
        tious diseases have been clinically excluded
Rapid (point of care) diagnostic testing (RDT)
Treatment protocols per local health authorities
Essential drugs
Referral guidelines
Secondary prevention
    community education
        health messages—printed, loudspeaker, broadcast, community groups
        community understands transmission and prevention measures

Epidemic Management

Outbreak management protocol
Secondary prevention
Resource prepositioning (stockpiles & supply chain management)
      indoor residual spraying (IRS) (within 2 weeks of epidemic)
            mass fever treatment (MFT) (active case finding & fever treatment with antimalarials)
            mass drug administration (MDA) (cover 80% of population within 2 weeks)
Information management
Contingency planning

Reference

1. Connolly, M. (Ed). (2005). *Communicable disease control in emergencies—a field manual.* Geneva: World Health Organization.

MEASLES

Preventive Medicine

EPI
Subnational immunization days
Measles immunization of contacts of confirmed case if contacts have < 2 doses of vaccine

Epidemiological Surveillance

Surveillance definition becomes clinical once outbreak is lab-confirmed

Clinical Medicine

Delivery of Health Services

Active case finding through CHWs

Standardized Case Management

Case definition
    An illness characterized by all of the following clinical features: a generalized rash lasting greater than or equal to 3 d (exanthems generally without symmetry or pruritis); $T \geq 38.3$ °C (101 °F); cough, or coryza, or conjunctivitis
Treatment protocols emphasizing supportive care and treatment of complications
    Vitamin A

Table 8.6.6
Vitamin A Treatment Schedules in Infant/Child Deficiency States

Age	Initial Dose	Next Day Dose
0–6 months	50,000 IU	50,000 IU
6–11 months	100,000 IU	100,000 IU
1+ years	200,000 IU	200,000 IU

Essential drugs
Referral guidelines
Secondary prevention
    community education
        health messages—printed, loudspeaker, broadcast, community groups
        community understands measles transmission and prevention measures

Epidemic Management

Identify cause of the outbreak
Undertake vaccination campaign
Strengthen routine immunization and surveillance

Table 8.6.7
Population Vaccination Status and Contributing Causes

Vaccination Status and Patient Age	Probably Cause
> 50% cases U5 & unvaccinated	low coverage
> 50% cases U5 & vaccinated	not measles or vaccine ineffective
> 50% cases O5 in high coverage area	disease shift to older age group
high % of cases in infants	low routine coverage

MENINGITIS

Pathogens and Epidemiology

Meningitis is a disease with significant mortality. Meningococcus (*Neisseria meningitides*) is renown for its rapid onset, rapid progression (death sometimes within hours), and high mortality (50% untreated).

There are 13 serogroups of *Neisseria meningitides* but only 6 (A, B, C, W, X, Y) are known to cause epidemics.

The bacteria spread from person to person via respiratory and nasal secretions. Kissing, sharing eating and drinking utensils, cigarettes, coughing, and sneezing are recognized methods of transmission. Close contacts over a period of time, as between household or dormitory residents, are most commonly affected. Population movements (e.g. pilgrimages, displacement, military recruitment), poor living conditions, and overcrowding are epidemic risk factors.

Large, recurring epidemics of meningitis occur in the "meningitis belt" of sub-Saharan Africa where over 430 million people live. This belt encompasses 26 countries from Senegal in the west to Ethiopia in the east and as far south as Tanzania and the Democratic Republic of Congo. Sub-saharan Arica has epidemic seasonality. Dry seasons and droughts favor epidemics. Rains stop them. Large regional epidemics, as well as epidemics in displaced populations and refugee camps, have mainly been due to meningococcus serogroup A. Since 2010, extensive use of meningococcal type A conjugate vaccine in the meningitis belt has reduced the incidence and case load of type A epidemics by nearly 60%. In 2016, the most common lab confirmed meningitis isolate was *Streptococcus pneumoniae*.

In non-epidemic settings, *Neisseria.meningitidis*, *Streptococcus pneumoniae*, and *Haemophilus influenzae* account for 80% of all cases of bacterial meningitis. Prior to the availability of conjugate vaccines, *H. influenza* type b (Hib) was the most common cause of childhood bacterial meningitis outside of epidemics. Where Hib vaccines are in the routine infant immunization schedule, Hib meningitis has nearly disappeared.

Preventive Medicine

Polysaccharide vaccines are available with 2 serotypes (A and C), 3 serotypes (A, C and W) or 4 serotypes (A,C, W, and Y). Duration of immunity is approximately 3 years.

Meningococcal protein conjugate vaccines confer longer immunity but at higher cost than polysaccharide vaccines. Monovalent conjugate vaccine against group C dates from 1999, and tetravalent (A, C, W and Y) conjugate vaccine dates from 2005. A group B vaccine made from 4 bacterial proteins has been licensed since 2014 but is not readily available.

Meningococcal vaccines have a very low incidence of side effects.

Epidemiological Surveillance

Regular disease surveillance is necessary to detect outbreaks. The epidemic threshold is 10 suspected cases/100,0000 population in any given week. Two suspected cases of meningitis in the same settlement should trigger an outbreak investigation.

Nasopharyngeal carriage rates do not predict epidemics.

Clinical Medicine

80–85% of meningococcal disease presents with meningitis. 80% of cases occur in patients < 30 y/o. Peak incidence in meningitis belt is ages 5–10 yrs. Diagnosis is straightforward when patient presents with signs of meningitis—fever, headache, vomiting, changes in mental status. However, most patients have non-specific illness 1–3 days before onset of meningitis. CFR of untreated meningococcal meningitis can be 50%. CFR of properly treated meningococcal meningitis is <1%.

15–20% of meningococcal disease presents with septicemia unaccompanied by meningitis or other focal features. It is a dramatic illness which affects previously healthy children and young adults. It presents with acute fever leading to purpura fulminans (hemorrhagic or purpuric rash), shock, and Waterhouse-Friderichsen syndrome (acute adrenal failure). Etiologic diagnosis can be easily missed. CFR of meningococcal septicemia is 50% and may be 25% even with proper treatment.

Diagnosis may be confirmed by agglutination tests, polymerase chain reaction, culture and sensitivity testing of spinal fluid and blood. In many situations, these tests are not available. Throat swabs may be helpful on occasions. **Do not delay treatment for tests or test results. Minutes count. It is more important to have a live patient without a confirmed diagnosis than a dead one with a diagnosis**.

Differential diagnosis in a tropical patient with fever and altered mental status, but without purpura or shock, includes cerebral malaria. Co-infection may occur.

Standardized case management of bacterial meningitis in developed countries involves 7–10 days of parenteral antibiotic therapy. Drug of choice in adults and older children is ceftriaxone which also rapidly eliminates the carrier state. Alternate drugs include ampicillin and benzylpenicillin which do not eliminate the carrier state. In developing countries, 4 days of parenteral antibiotic therapy are empirically shown to be effective. In large epidemics in resource-poor settings, a single IM dose of chloramphenicol in oil is the drug of choice. For patients who do not improve in 48 h, a repeat dose may be given.

Viral meningitis is rarely serious and requires only supportive care, Recovery is usually complete.

Patient isolation and disinfection of the room, clothing, or bedding are not necessary. Respiratory precautions are advised particularly early in the course of treatment.

Chemoprophylaxis of contacts is available in some settings but rarely in the disaster setting. Vigilance and education of close contacts is mandatory.

Epidemic Management

Epidemic preparedness and early detection of outbreaks are key.

Vaccines against *N. meningitides* serogroups A, C, Y and W135 are very effective in controlling epidemics. In epidemic settings, children 2–10 are the priority target with serogroups A and C typically the priority antigens. Rapid mass vaccination campaigns can contain outbreaks in 2–3 weeks. For immunocompetent patients over 2 years, vaccine efficacy rate is 90% one week after injection. However, duration of immunity may be as little as 2 years in younger children. In some countries, vaccine may also be used with close contacts of sporadic disease cases to prevent secondary cases.

Chemoprophylaxis of contacts is not recommended in epidemics, but community education and ready access to health care are essential.

VIRAL HEMORRHAGIC FEVER

Preventive Medicine

Source control/reduction/elimination

>Avoid unnecessary contact with suspected reservoir animals and known disease carrier species (e.g. primates).
>
>Avoid direct or close contact with symptomatic patients.
>
>Undertake quarantine and culling of sick reservoir animals and known disease carrier species.
>
>Avoid unnecessary contact with or consumption of dead reservoir animals or known disease carrier species.
>
>Establish appropriate communicable disease controls for burial of the dead.

Administrative controls

Environmental and engineering controls

>Avoid needle stick exposure to blood specimens thru automated machine handling

PPE

>Use standard precautions—gloves, masks, and protective clothing—if handling infected animals or patients.
>
>Wash hands after visiting sick patients.

Epidemiological Surveillance

Active surveillance and contact tracing (enhanced surveillance) through community-based mobile teams

Clinical Medicine

Delivery of Health Services

Active case finding (screening and triage) and contact tracing

Dedicated isolation facility

Food provision to isolated patients so they are not dependent on family

Standardized Case Management

Case definition

Treatment protocols emphasizing supportive care and treatment of complications

Essential drugs

Referral guidelines

Secondary prevention

>barrier nursing strictly enforced
>
>family and community education

Epidemic Management

Ministerial task force to address policy

Local health authority task force to address procedures

National level task forces to comprise

>Response unit
>
>>epidemiology (case finding, contact tracing, monitoring, surveillance)
>>
>>facilities preparation (build beds)
>>
>>case management
>>
>>laboratory
>>
>>infection prevention and control (IPC) (including safe burial)
>>
>>social mobilization, communication
>>
>>training
>
>Support unit (manage resources)
>
>>program & HR planning (16 positions)
>>
>>staffing model

1. social/medical/cultural anthropologist
2. social mobilization/community engagement specialist
3. social mobilization coordinator at national level
4. epidemiologist
5. IPC specialist
6. PH advisor
7. subnational field coordinator
8. VHF lab specialist
9. case management specialist
10. EMTs
11. occupational health and safety specialist
12. logistics
13. exit screening
14. data management
15. health communications
16. finance

Research unit
    new therapeutics
    new tests
    clinical trials
    analytic epi and modelling

Long term measures
    health systems recovery

Outbreak management in the field focuses on
    alert verification
    disease surveillance (not relying exclusively or even largely on health facility reporting)
    burial < 48 h after death
    spot checking of contact tracing effectiveness (< 5 is inadequate; 25–50 is reasonable; 75 is not extreme)
    door-to-door community education campaigns
    quarantine sustainment at HH level

Secondary prevention

Resource prepositioning (stockpiles & supply chain management)

Information management—refute inappropriate travel and trade restrictions

Community education and social mobilization
    health messages—printed, loudspeaker, broadcast, community groups
    community understands disease transmission and prevention measures

Contingency planning

NB   it's difficult to separate ebola from non-ebola fevers at onset
       holding centers can amplify transmission

Annex 8.7
DIAGNOSTIC LABORATORY IN INFECTIOUS DISEASES

Glossary

Ab	antibody
AFB	acid-fast bacilli
Ag	antigen
C&S	culture and antibiotic sensitivity
CIE	counterimmunoelectrophoresis
COTS	Cholera Outbreak Training and Shigellosis Program (training program developed at ICDDR)
CSF	cerebrospinal fluid
ELISA	enzyme-linked immunosorbent assay
d	day
HAI	hemagglutination inhibition
IgG, IgM	immunoglobulin G, M
O&P	ova and parasite (stool slide examination)
PCR	polymerase chain reaction
Pt	patient
RDT	rapid diagnostic test
TB	tuberculosis

Lab Purposes

- Confirm syndromic or clinical diagnosis
  - Identify treatment options
  - Identify control measures
- Characterize the agent (serotype, biotype, antibiogram, etc.)
  - Evaluate potential effectiveness of treatment
  - Monitor the spread of a particular clone or subtype
- Detect an outbreak and confirm its end

Key Questions on Lab (WHO [1])

1. Is a laboratory available?
2. What tests does it perform?
3. Is there transport to and from the laboratory?
4. Who prepares transport media?
5. Who provides specimen collection material and supplies?
6. How can these supplies be obtained?
7. Who provides cool packs, transport boxes, car, driver …?
8. What forms/information must be sent with the specimens?
9. What epidemiological information must accompany test results?
10. How does the epidemiologist obtain results?

If a lab is not available, then you need a sampling strategy that addresses specimen acquisition, preparation, and transportation in compliance with international regulations on the transport of infetious substances.

Table 8.7.1
Indications, Laboratory Tests, and Expected Availability

Cases	Lab tests	PHC clinic	Confirmation laboratory
Watery diarrhea—dehydrating (suspected cholera)	• Fine microscopy for motility on wet prep, O&P	• +	• District lab
	• Gram's stain	• +	• District lab
	• Stool C&S	• +/−	• District lab
	• Toxin or polysaccharide (RDT)	• ?	• District lab
Diarrhea with blood (shigella, salmonella, amoeba)	• Fine microscopy for O&P	• +	• District lab
	• Stool C&S	• +/−	• District lab
Acute respiratory infection	• Strep screen, throat C&S	• +	• District lab
	• Microscopy with Ziehl-Neelsen stain for AFB	• +	• District lab
Acute febrile illness (suspected malaria)	• Microscopy with Giemsa stain	• +	• District lab
	• Ag detection (RDT)	• +	• District lab
Acute febrile illness (suspected typhoid)	• Blood culture	• -	• District lab
	• Serology (ELISA, RDT)	• -	• District lab
Meningitis (suspected meningococcus)	• CSF microscopy with Gram's stain	• +	• District lab
	• CSF C&S	• −	• District lab
	• CSF PCR	• −	• District lab
Acute jaundice syndrome (suspected viral hepatitis)	• Serology	• −	• District lab
Acute flaccid paralysis (suspected poliomyelitis)	• Virus isolation (cell culture from stool specimens)	• −	• Reference lab
Measles	• Serology (IgM)	None—clinical Dx	• District lab
Neonatal tetanus	None—clinical Dx	None—clinical Dx	None—clinical Dx
Acute febrile illness (suspected influenza)	• Ag detection (RDT—Types A, B)	• ?	• District lab
	• PCR	• −	• District lab
Acute febrile illness (suspected dengue fever)	• Ab detection (RDT) immunochromatography	• −	• District lab
	• Serology (IgM of paired sera)	• −	• District lab
	• PCR	• −	• Reference lab
Leptospirosis	• Ab detection (RDT)	• −	• Reference lab
	• Serology (ELISA)	• −	• Reference lab
Typhus	• Serology	• −	• Reference lab

Direct techniques

    microscopy (direct visualization)

    culture (isolation)

    immunological Ag techniques—immunochromatography, latex agglutination (vibrio)

    molecular Ag techniques—DNA or RNA PCR, antigen capture

Indirect serological (Ab) techniques

    bacterial agglutination

    hemagglutination inhibition assay

    ELISA for IgM, IgG

    microneutralization assay

    NB   no specific response from some organisms; little or no response in immunosuppression delays in serological response oblige testing of early and late sera

Table 8.7.2
Specimen Handling (adapted from WHO [1])

Clinical Syndrome and Lab Details

Early stages of infection, during peaks of fever, and before ABX

Issue				
When to sample?	• acute diarrhea • acute flaccid paralysis	• meningitis	• fevers • icterus • measles	• misc
What to sample?	• stool	• cerebrospinal fluid	• whole blood	• sputum for TB • urine for schisto, lepto • bubo aspirate for plague
How many samples and how often to sample?	• 10–20 samples (different Pts) initially to confirm outbreak • 10–20 samples each month to verify strain and drug susceptibility (systematic random sampling with skip interval of monthly total visits/sample size) • 10–20 samples (different Pts) after epidemic to confirm resolution (COTS avoids this as cholera or shigella usually causes < 5% of all diarrhea outside of epidemic)		• 10 samples initially, but strategy may vary with disease • paired samples for serology—early and after 7–14 d	
Biosafety while sampling?	• protect yourself (universal precautions, personal protective equipment as needed) • protect the Pt (disinfect, use single use materials) • protect the environment (waste disposal, triple package the specimen)			
How to sample?	• collect liquid stool in leak-proof container • use forceps to immerse swab or filter paper dots in liquid stool; place in specimen container with a few drops of sterile saline • for bloody stool, sample several areas of specimen including blood, mucous, or tissue	• lumbar puncture in usual way	• venipuncture in usual way	
How to prepare the sample?	• Cary Blair* • Trans Isolate (cost high) • Alcaline peptone water (if < 6 h before plating) • saline solution	• Trans Isolate⁺	• whole blood for CBC, microscopy (purple cap—EDTA tube) • serum for serology (red cap—no additive; orange cap—gel separator) • whole blood for blood culture (biphasic culture bottle—10% blood to media ratio) obtain before starting ABX • blood smear for malaria microscopy	

Clinical Syndrome and Lab Details

Issue				
How to preserve and send the sample?	• refrigerate if possible (4° C) or cool packs	• incubate Trans Isolate for culture (25–37 °C) • refrigerate other vials for cytology, chemistry (4° C)	• incubate blood culture (25–37° C) • refrigerate sera (4-8°C) • ambient temp for smears	• refrigerate specimen (4° C)
	Triple package in appropriate packaging (e.g. local official container or consistent with international regulation 650) 1. leak-proof specimen container wrapped with enough absorbent material to absorb the entire content of the 1st container 2. leak-proof secondary container usually plastic or metal 3. outer shipping container whose smallest dimension is 10mm Diagnostic specimens use IATA packing instruction 650 without biohazard label. Infectious materials use IATA packing instruction 602 with biohazard label.			
What to send with the sample?	Lab request form with: • sender's name and contact info • patient name, age, sex • sample date, time • suspected clinical diagnosis with main signs and symptoms • sample macroscopic description • context—outbreak confirmation, ongoing verification, outbreak end, etc. • epidemiological or demographic data			
Where to send the sample?	• reference lab • contact person			
What and when to expect results?				

Source: World Health Organization. Highlights of specimen collection in emergency situations. Undated. Used with permission of WHO.

* Semi-solid transport medium, easy to use
Place swab with sample in medium to immerse tip of swab. Break off wooden swab handle. Cap tightly.
Use with stool and other samples containing non-fragile bacterial pathogens.
Inexpensive medium. Long shelf life after preparation (about 1 year at 25 °C). Can be prepared in advance and pre-positioned at peripheral levels.

\+ Biphasic transport medium with agar and broth
Pre-warm medium to 25–37 °C before inoculation. Place 1 cc of specimen in sterile medium for culture. Immediately incubate or hold at 25–37 °C. Ventilate bottle if > 4 days to lab.
Place 1 cc of specimen in another sterile vial for cytology, chemistry, and CIE. Refrigerate.
More expensive medium.

Reference

1. World Health Organization Department of Communicable Disease Surveillance and Response. *Highlights of specimen collection in emergency situations*. Undated. Available from WHO Laboratory and Epidemiology Capacity Strengthening Office in Lyon, France, and Retrieved June 9, 2017, from http://www.who.int/hac/techguidance/training/highlights%20of%20specimen%20collection_en.pdf.

Annex 8.8
ACRONYMS

ABC	abstain until marriage, be faithful, use condoms
ACAPS	Assessment Capacities Project
ACT	artemisinin-based combination therapy
ADB	Asian Development Bank
AfDB	African Development Bank Group
AFRO	Africa Regional Office (WHO)
AI	avian influenza
AIDS	acquired immune deficiency syndrome
AKF	Aga Khan Foundation
ALDAC	all diplomatic and consular posts (USG)
ALNAP	Active Learning Network for Accountability and Performance (ODI)
AMB E&P	Ambassador Extraordinary and Plenipotentiary
AMRO	Americas Regional Office (WHO)
APS	annual program statement (USAID\OFDA statement of funding opportunities for NGOs)
APW	agreement for the performance of work (WHO contractual work agreement)
ARI	acute respiratory infection
ART	antiretroviral therapy
AU	African Union
BCC	behavior change communication
BCP	business continuity planning
BIC	basic internet communications
BMS	breast milk substitute
BSL	biosafety security level
BWI	Bretton Woods Institutions (World Bank and International Monetary Fund)
CA	cooperative agreement
CAP	consolidated appeals process (supplanted in 2013 by the humanitarian programme cycle; led by OCHA)
CBJ	Congressional budget justification
CBO	community-based organization
CBPF	country-based pooled funds (amalgamation of Emergency Response Funds and Common Humanitarian Funds administered by OCHA)
CBRNE	chemical, biological, radiological, nuclear, or explosive
CCCM	camp coordination and camp management
CCS	country cooperation strategy (WHO)
CCTV	closed-circuit television
CD	communicable diseases
CDC	communicable disease control; Centers for Disease Control and Prevention (US)
CE	complex emergency
CERF	Central Emergency Response Fund (administered by OCHA)
CFE	Contingency Fund for Emergencies (WHO)
CHW	community health worker
CLA	cluster lead agency
CMAM	community-based management of acute malnutrition
CMOC	civil-military operations center
CMR	crude mortality rate
CO	country office (WHO)
COD	common operational dataset
CoDel	Congressional Delegation
COG	continuity of government
CONOPS	concept of operations
CoOp	continuity of operations

COP	common operating picture
CPA	comprehensive peace agreement
CRED	Center for Research on the Epidemiology of Disasters (Belgium)
CSP	certified safety professional
CSW	commercial sex worker
CTC	community therapeutic care (of malnutrition)
CTO	cognizant technical officer
CTP	cash transfer program
DA	development assistance—US Congress appropriated funds with tight reporting requirements
DANIDA	Danish International Development Agency
DART	Disaster Assistance Response Team (USAID)
DCHA	Bureau for Democracy, Conflict, and Humanitarian Assistance (USAID)
DDR(P)	disarmament, demobilization, and reintegration program
DDRR(P)	disarmament, demobilization, rehabilitation, and reintegration program
DDRRR(P)	disarmament, demobilization, repatriation, resettlement, and reintegration program
DFID	Department for International Development (UK)
DHN	digital humanitarian network
DHO	District Health Office
DMAT	Disaster Medical Assistance Team (US)
DMORT	Disaster Mortuary Operational Response Team
DO	designated official (UN)
DOD	Department of Defense (US)
DOS	Department of State (US)
DOTS	direct observed therapy short-course (used for TB)
DRM	disaster risk management
DRR	disaster risk reduction
DS	diplomatic security
DTM	displacement tracking matrix
ECHO	European Community Humanitarian Office (European Commission Directorate General for Humanitarian Aid and Civil Protection which uses ECHO acronym)
EDG	Emergency Directors' Group
EHK	emergency health kit
EIA	environmental impact assessment
EMRO	Eastern Mediterranean Regional Office (WHO)
EMS	Emergency Medical Services
EMT	Emergency Medical Team
EOC	Emergency Operations Center
EOD	explosive ordnance disposal
EPI	Expanded Programme on Immunization
ERC	Emergency Relief Coordinator (UN)
ERF	Emergency Response Framework (WHO)
ERT	Emergency Response Team (WHO)
ESF	emergency school feeding
EST	Emergency Support Team (WHO)
EU	European Union
EURO	European Regional Office (WHO)
EWAR, EWS	early warning system
EWARN	Early Warning Alert and Response Network
FACT	Field Assessment Coordination Team (IFRC)
FAO	Food and Agriculture Organization (UN)
FCV	fragility, conflict, and violence
FEMA	Federal Emergency Management Agency (US)
FETP	Field Epidemiology Training Program

FEWS	Famine Early Warning Systems
FEWS NET	Famine Early Warning Systems Network
FFA	food assistance for assets (formerly food for work)
FFP	Food for Peace (USAID\DCHA office)
FOG	*Field Operations Guide* (OFDA)
FSN	foreign service national
FSO	field security officer
FTS	Financial Tracking Service (OCHA)
FY	fiscal year
G 8	group of 8 countries
G 20	group of 20 countries
G 77	group of 77 countries
GAM	global acute malnutrition (moderate + severe acute malnutrition)
GBV	gender-based violence
GDACS	Global Disaster Alert and Coordination System
GDP	gross domestic product
GEMT	Global Emergency Management Team (WHO)
GFATM	Global Fund to Fight AIDS, Tuberculosis and Malaria
GFD	general food distribution
GFDDR	Global Facility for Disaster Reduction and Recovery (WBG)
GHC	Global Health Cluster
GHD	good humanitarian donorship (initiated by DFID)
GHSA	Global Health Security Agenda
GIC	Global Impact Charities (consortium of faith-based organizations involved in HA)
GIEWS	Global Information and Early Warning System (FAO)
GIS	geographic information system
GNP	gross national product
GO	governmental organization
GOARN	Global Outbreak Alert and Response Network
GPN	global private network
GTZ	German Technical Cooperation
HA	humanitarian assistance
HAART	highly active anti-retroviral treatment
HAZMAT	hazardous materials
HBP	Health as a Bridge for Peace (WHO headquarters program initiative, now discontinued)
HC	Humanitarian Coordinator (IASC)
HCC	Health Cluster Coordinator
HCT	Humanitarian Country Team
HCW	health care worker
HDR	humanitarian daily ration
HELP	Health Emergencies in Large Populations (ICRC training course)
HEPA	high efficiency particulate aspirator (air filter)
HeRAMS	Health Resources Availability and Mapping System
HEWS	Humanitarian Early Warning System
HH	household
HHA	humanitarian health assistance
HHS	Department of Health and Human Services (US)
HIC	Humanitarian Information Centre (OCHA)
HIS	health information system
HIU	Humanitarian Information Unit (US DOS)
HIV	human immunodeficiency virus
HNO	humanitarian needs overview
HOA	Head of Office

HPAI	highly pathogenic avian influenza
HPC	humanitarian programme cycle
HPF	humanitarian pooled fund
HRP	humanitarian response plan (akin to SRP)
HWCO	Head of WHO Country Office
IAHE	interagency humanitarian evaluation (IASC process, triggered by L3 declaration, to be done within 12 m of declaration)
IAP	incident action plan
IASC	Interagency Standing Committee
IATA	International Air Transport Association
IBRD	International Bank for Reconstruction and Development (World Bank)
ICC	International Criminal Court
ICCG	Intercluster Coordination Group
ICDDR	International Centre for Diarrhoeal Disease Research, Bangladesh
ICMH	International Centre for Migration and Health
ICRC	International Committee of the Red Cross
ICS	Incident Command System
ID	infectious disease
IDA	International Development Association
IDFA	international disaster and famine account—US Congress appropriated funds which have no Congressional Note reporting requirements (see DA)
IDLH	immediately dangerous to life and health
IDP	internally displaced person
IDSR	Integrated Disease Surveillance and Response (AFRO initiative expanded to other regions)
IDU	injection drug user
IEC	information, education, and communication materials
IED	improvised explosive device
IEIP	International Emerging Infections Programs—foreign centers of excellence working in partnership with domestic MOH and US CDC which train local scientists, provide diagnostic and epi resources in outbreaks, and undertake regional disease control activities
IFRC	International Federation of Red Cross and Red Crescent Societies
IGS	income generating scheme
IHL	international humanitarian law
IHR	International Health Regulations
IHRL	international human rights law
ILI	influenza-like illness
IMAI	Integrated Management of Adult Illness (WHO initiative)
IMCI	Integrated Management of Childhood Illness (WHO initiative)
IMF	International Monetary Fund
IMS	incident management system
INSARAG	International Search and Rescue Advisory Group
IO	international organization
IOM	International Organization for Migration
IPC	Integrated Food Security Phase Classification
IRA	initial rapid assessment
IRC	International Rescue Committee
IRIN	Integrated Regional Information Network (OCHA)
ISDR	International Strategy for Disaster Reduction
ITN	insecticide treated nets
ITPS	insecticide treated plastic sheeting
ITWL	insecticide treated wall lining
IYCFE	infant and young child feeding in emergencies
JICA	Japan International Cooperation Agency

L3	level 3 (system-wide) emergency
LOU	letter of understanding
M&E	monitoring and evaluation
MCH	maternal and child health
MCI	mass casualty incident
MDGs	millennium development goals (supplanted by sustainable development goals)
MDM	Médecins du Monde
MDRO	Mission Disaster Relief Officer (USAID)
MEAL	monitoring, evaluation, accountability, and learning
MEB	minimum expenditure basket
MEDS	minimum essential datasets
MICS	multiple indicator cluster survey
MIRA	multi-cluster initial rapid assessment
MIS	management information system
MISP	minimum initial service package (used in reproductive health)
MOH	Ministry of Health
MOSS	minimum operating security standards (UNDSS)
MOU	memorandum of understanding
MSF	Médecins sans Frontières
MUAC	mid-upper arm circumference
NAF	needs analysis framework
NATO	North Atlantic Treaty Organization
NDMA	National Disaster Management Agency
NDMS	National Disaster Medical System (US)
NFI	non-food item (emergency relief supplies)
NGO	non-governmental organization
NIC	National Influenza Center
NICS	nutritional information in crisis situations
NID	national immunization day
NIH	National Institutes of Health (US)
NIMA	National Imagery and Mapping Agency (US)
NRC	Norwegian Refugee Council
NRF	National Response Framework (US)
NSS	National Security Staff (US)
NZODA	New Zealand Official Development Assistance
OCHA	Office for the Coordination of Humanitarian Affairs (UN)
ODI	Overseas Development Institute (UK)
OECD	Organization for Economic Cooperation and Development
OFDA	Office of US Foreign Disaster Assistance (USAID)
OHCHR	Office of the High Commissioner for Human Rights (UN)
OI	opportunistic infection
OIE	Office International des Epizooties (World Organization for Animal Health)
OPD	outpatient department
OPR	operational peer review (IASC process, triggered by L3 declaration, to be done within 90 d of declaration)
ORS	oral rehydration salts/solution
OSCE	Office for Security and Cooperation in Europe
OSOCC	On-Site Operations Coordination Center (UN)
OVC	orphans and vulnerable children
PAHO	Pan-American Health Organization (precursor to and functionally synonymous with AMRO)
PDD	Presidential Decision Directive
PDNA	post-disaster needs assessment
PEF	Pandemic Emergency Financing Facility (WBG)

PEP	post-exposure prophylaxis
PEPFAR	President's Emergency Plan for AIDS Relief (US)
PHC	primary health care
PHEIC	public health event of international concern (IHR)
PHO	Provincial Health Office
PIO	public international organization
PKO	peace-keeping organization
PLWHA	person living with HIV/AIDS
PMTCT	prevention of mother-to-child transmission
PNG	persona non grata
POC	point of contact
POLR	provider of last resort
POW	prisoner of war
PPE	personal protective equipment
PPM	parts per million = mg/L (1 ppm = 1mg/L = .0001% active ingredient)
PPRR	prevention, preparedness, response, and recovery
PRA	participatory rural appraisal (successor to the RRA)
PRRA	participatory rapid rural appraisal
PSC	personal services contractor
PSD	protective security detail
PSF	Pharmaciens Sans Frontières
PVO	private and voluntary organization
R2D	relief to development
R2P	responsibility to protect
R4	repatriation, reintegration, rehabilitation, and reconstruction
R&R	rest and recreation
RBM	Roll Back Malaria (WHO program)
RC	Resident Coordinator (UN)
REA	rapid epidemiological assessment
RFA	request for assistance
RFI	request for information
RFP	request for proposal
RFQ	request for quote
RH	reproductive health
RMO	Regional Medical Officer (US Department of State)
RMT	Response Management Team (USAID)
RNI	recommended nutritional intake (successor to the recommended daily allowance (RDA))
RO	regional office
RRA	rapid rural appraisal; rapid response account (WHO)
RRM	rapid response mechanism
RRT	rapid response team
RSO	Regional Security Officer (US Department of State)
RUSF	ready-to-use supplementary food
RUTF	ready-to-use therapeutic food
SAR	search and rescue
SARS	severe acute respiratory syndrome
SBU	sensitive but unclassified
SC	Security Council (UN)
SCF	Save the Children Foundation
SCI	secret compartmented information
SDGs	sustainable development goals
SEARO	South-East Asia Regional Office (WHO)
SFC	supplementary feeding center

SFP	supplemental feeding program
SGBV	sexual and gender-based violence
SHOC	Strategic Health Operations Center (WHO)
SMART	Standardized Monitoring and Assessment of Relief and Transitions
SME	subject matter expert
SMS	Security Management System (UN)
SMT	Security Management Team (UN)
SNS	Strategic National Stockpile (US)
SO	strategic objective (> 5 yrs to achieve)
SOD	sudden onset disaster
SOG	standard operating guideline
SOP	standard operating procedure
SPHC	selective primary health care
SPHERE	project of humanitarian agencies detailing a humanitarian charter and minimum standards
SpO	special objective (< 5 yrs to achieve)
SRP	strategic response plan
SRSG	Special Representative of the Secretary General (UN)
STI	sexually transmitted infection
SUMA	supply management (PAHO/WHO program)
SWAP	sector-wide approach
TAG	Technical Assistance Group (USAID\OFDA)
TB	tuberculosis
TBA	traditional birth attendant
TFC	therapeutic feeding center
TFP	therapeutic feeding program
TOR	terms of reference
UMDMT	UN Disaster Management Team
UN	United Nations
UNAIDS	Joint United Nations AIDS Programme
UNCT	UN Country Team
UNDAC	UN Disaster Assessment and Coordination team
UNDAF	UN Development Assistance Framework
UNDP	UN Development Programme
UNDPKO	UN Department of Peacekeeping Operations
UNDSS	UN Department of Safety and Security
UNEP	UN Environmental Programme
UNFPA	UN Fund for Population Activities
UNGA	UN General Assembly
UNHAS	UN Humanitarian Air Service (WFP)
UNHCHR	UN High Commissioner for Human Rights
UNHCR	UN High Commissioner for Refugees
UNHRD	UN Humanitarian Response Depot
UNICEF	UN Children's Fund
UNJLC	UN Joint Logistics Center
UNPKO	UN Peace-keeping Operations
UNRC	UN Resident Coordinator
UNSE	UN Special Envoy
UNSG	UN Secretary General
UNV	UN volunteer
USAID	US Agency for International Development
USAR	urban search and rescue
USCR	US Committee for Refugees
USD	US dollar

USDA	US Department of Agriculture
USG	Under Secretary General (UN); US Government
USPHS	US Public Health Service
UXO	unexploded ordnance
VAC	Vulnerability Assessment Committee
VAM	vulnerability assessment and mapping (WFP)
VCT	voluntary counseling and testing (HIV)
WASH	water, sanitation, and hygiene
WBG	World Bank Group
WCO	WHO Country Office
WFP	World Food Programme (UN)
WHE	WHO Health Emergencies Programme
WHO	World Health Organization (UN)
WHZ	weight-for-height z score
WMD	weapons of mass destruction
WPRO	Western Pacific Regional Office (WHO)
WR	WHO Representative (replaced by HWCO)
WWWW, 4W	who does what where when (matrix)

Contents

Guidance Notes

This section addresses resilience in the field and reentry on repatriation. There is a burgeoning literature on these subjects in the general context of staff wellness. Organizations take increasing responsibility for it, and their guidance is increasingly authoritative. The challenge for the responder is to develop a robust personal resilience strategy before deployment and a reentry strategy before return.

Resilience Checklist (Document 9.1)

Resilience has physical and psychological components. These components can be embedded in a series of "schedules" for activities of daily living in disaster. Seven "schedules" are particularly relevant—work, sleep, eating, exercise, recreation, socialization, and meditation. Comments on implementation technique follow below.

- **Work**
  Security conditions may force you into irregular and extended work schedules. Prepare to work over 80 h/week. The science of chronobiology can help mitigate the challenges of jet lag and shift changes on-site.
- **Sleep**
  Cool ambient temperatures, noise cancellation/control, parasympathetic induction, and tryptophan loading are useful adjuncts. Ultimately, a big decision occurs at 1:00 AM when you must be functional in the morning, have a 4 h sleep window before roosters, road traffic, and call to prayer awaken you, and none of the foregoing adjuncts are helping. In situations where you are not "on-call" through the night, a short-acting benzodiazepine (e.g., triazolam) can be useful. Air force pilots with 4 h downtime between serial sorties have used short-acting benzos to sleep with no appreciable degradation of subsequent psychomotor performance. These drugs must be trialed before deployment to ensure familiarity with therapeutic effect and absence of untoward side effects. Limit PRN drug taking. After 3–4 weeks of nocturnal use, you will experience interrupted sleep on drug cessation.

© David A. Bradt 2019
D. A. Bradt, C. M. Drummond, *Reference Manual for Humanitarian Health Professionals*,
https://doi.org/10.1007/978-3-319-69871-7_9

- **Eating**

  Get to like pulses and starches. Figure out what you can do to make them appetizing for months at a time. Try to limit intake of provocative agents—alcohol, caffeine, tobacco, and sugar. In some cultures, this can be difficult. Moreover, try not to let individual dietary preferences become a team issue. Macrobiotic vegans who insist on dietary adherence but lack self-sufficiency become a nuisance to the team.

- **Exercise**

  There are many dimensions to exercise—strength, stamina, speed, endurance, flexibility, power, coordination, agility, balance, and accuracy. The best routines incorporate all these dimensions. Selected adjuncts can be useful—stretch belts, yoga pads, etc. Relevant items belong on a packing list insofar as resilience can be planned. More spartan, and probably more useful, are empty hand martial art techniques—e.g., kata, kihon, kumite—which require no equipment, no partner, and little space.

- **Recreation**

  This schedule overlaps with exercise, but it encompasses many non-exertional activities as well—reading, playing games, playing music, listening to music, etc. Find an activity you enjoy which keeps you from ruminating on dramas of the day and helps rejuvenate you.

- **Socialization**

  Be relaxed but purposeful, here. It's easy to retreat from socializing in favor of other duties. However, socialization should be treated as part of your cocoon of safety. The people who handle your comms, security, and medevac can save your life, and you can contribute to their cocoon of safety as well.

- **Meditation**

  Effective techniques may be applied in the field, but mastery begins at home well before deployment. Deep breathing, progressive muscle relaxation, and color imagery are enabling steps. Auto-induced bradycardia is an excellent marker of autonomic control. Athletic conditioning and stimulus desensitization can enhance mastery here.

All these schedules may be difficult to implement in the hyperacute phase of a sudden onset disaster or the exacerbated phase of a complex disaster. Individual schedules may be difficult to sustain over the course of any disaster. Nonetheless, each individual schedule contributes to personal resilience, and its effect can be synergistic—diet fuels exercise, exercise contributes to sleep quality, sleep quality contributes to work quality, etc. Moreover, intact schedules among the seven can mitigate the effects of interruption to other schedules.

The challenges of working in a disaster are predictable. The compensations and consequences can be uproariously funny. Conversely, some environments are so hostile and some consequences are so severe that survival itself is a success. You need to fully assess your hazardscape. If hostile environments are part of your duty station, than the need for survival skills emerges. Selected references for lethal situation management are listed below [1–4]. Survival tactics and training are beyond the scope of this *Manual* but not beyond the scope of your due diligence.

Reentry Checklist (Document 9.2)

Reentry can be the hardest part of the mission. Our experiences change us. Your insight to disaster ground truth will heighten awareness of (limits to) field security, communications, transport, environmental health, public services, clinical care, household vulnerability, and donor engagement. Your heightened awareness may be totally out of sync with the priorities and values of the society you reenter. The disconnect can be disturbing. "Stranger theory" has explored these issues in many social groups including displaced populations, diplomatic personnel, foreign exchange students, and development professionals. Disaster relief can also have a polarizing effect on people you meet. It can elicit plaudits and hero worship as well as condemnation and retribution. Recognize that reentry is an issue for all repatriating staff. You are likely to go thru it tired, jet lagged, distracted, irritable, and perhaps intolerant—the antithesis of resilient. Nonetheless, recognize the stakes are high. Collateral damage in a poorly executed reentry can adversely affect yourself, your family, and your friends. Hence, reentry deserves the same attention to detail as deployment.

References

1. Roberts, D. L. (2005). *Staying alive—Safety and security guidelines for humanitarian volunteers in conflict areas.* Geneva: International Committee of the Red Cross.
2. Gonzales, L. (2003). *Deep survival.* London: WW Norton & Co.
3. de Becker, G. (1997). *The gift of fear.* New York: Dell Publishing.
4. Fisher, R., & Ury, W. (1997). *Getting to yes—Negotiating agreement without giving in.* London: Arrow Books Limited.

Document 9.1
RESILIENCE CHECKLIST

A.   Preparedness

1.   Understand the seven schedules of resilience—work, sleep, eating, exercise, recreation, socialization, and meditation.
2.   Practice techniques to develop mastery over the schedules—particularly for sleep, exercise, and meditation.
3.   Understand the three step genesis of accidents and injuries—risky conditions, faulty judgment, and unsafe acts.
4.   Understand the differences between flameout, burnout, and post-traumatic stress. These stress reactions have vastly different therapeutic implications.
5.   Read the experience of your predecessors. *Deep Survival* and *The Gift of Fear* are core content.
6.   Think of rejuvenating activities you can do in the field. Pack items that may assist—list of exercises, adjuncts (e.g., stretch belts, exercise mat), small musical instrument, DVDs, cards, books.
7.   Work out the ABCs of stress management YOU will do in a hyperacute situation.

B.   On Mission

1.   Remember that team safety and security are the first priorities and may preempt attention to other issues.
2.   Rehearse the plans and skills in lethal situation management. Familiarity creates confidence and competence.
3.   Establish a buddy system within the team. It is a fundamental strategy in group safety and security, and affirms expectations that reaching out to each other is important.
4.   Be aware of other members of your team and how they are faring. Consider task team assignments and periodic socialization to help build esprit de corps and maintain resilience.
5.   Bond with people who have mastered the craft. They can change your life, and may even save it.
6.   Make new friends among the locals. They are your early warning system. Learn a few key words of the local language.
7.   Try to allocate time each day for your resilience activities. Avoid routines in high threat areas, but incorporate resilience activities into your daily schedule even if only for a few minutes.
8.   Learn stress management techniques you can do unobtrusively during the day and in your chair. Find time for relaxation activities before sleep. Engage in activities you found relaxing at home.
9.   Prioritize your work. Learn to say no to things that are not priority tasks. Focus on the things that only you can do. Delegate tasks as appropriate.
10.   When you have little experience with a new situation, learn to ask insightful questions and seek relevant counsel. The practice affirms the mindset that you don't have to have all the answers, but are smart enough to find them. The practice also makes it easier for you to reach out when issues become personal.
11.   Impulse control—observing, measuring, and thinking—may be the best initial response to a crisis situation.
12.   Beware of sexual contacts and promiscuity. Sex with team members, locals, prostitutes, or beneficiaries has progressive moral hazard and legal consequence. You can end up with HIV, without a job, and in jail.
13.   Stay positive and control your thoughts. Negativity is both a poison and an infectious disease.
14.   Minimize alcohol and avoid illicit drugs.
15.   Learn to tell a joke. Jokes on you are the best.
16.   When things are bad, take them 1 day at a time. When things are really bad, take them 5 minutes at a time. Stay alert, control your breathing, think clearly, and act decisively.
17.   Talk through bad news with someone you like and trust.
18.   Seek beauty in your environment. The stars at night are beautiful even if you are surrounded by death and destruction.
19.   Try not to lose your compassion.

Document 9.2
REENTRY CHECKLIST

A. Field Exit

1. A briefing book for your successor takes days to prepare. See Medical Handover Checklist in Sect. 2. Try to compile it incrementally instead of waiting until your end-of-mission.
2. Try to complete your end-of-mission report in the field. You don't want to bring back homework from the field. Try to get your report in early to colleagues with whom you will debrief.
3. Inform your field counterparts of your upcoming departure, make courtesy rounds with significant decision-makers, and leave them a token of esteem. You may never see them again, but your successor will inherit the relationship.
4. Try to debrief with your successor in the field, with your country office, and with your headquarters. You will be lucky if you get 2 out of 3.
5. Try to schedule regional R&R before you leave the field. Regional World Heritage Sites are well-worth visiting, and post-disaster hotel rates away from the relief community are never cheaper.

B. Reentry Home

1. Schedule plenty of rest and relaxation on your return. Avoid going straight back to work.
2. Don't over-program your days. You will probably have acute jet lag and chronic sleep debt.
3. Try not to make a significant decision or undertake a life event immediately on your return.
4. Try not to schedule yourself for clinical duties on your return. Admin, teaching, and research duties will generally be less demanding.
5. If you feel sick, seek a primary care provider or travel clinic. If you feel quite ill (high fever, rigor, malaise), seek a hospital emergency department. Do not delay. Tell them where you been been and request a work-up for endemic pathogens—malaria, occult bacteremia, arboviral disease, etc.
6. Don't expect your intimate partner to understand what you did in the field.
7. Don't expect your family and social friends to understand what you did in the field.
8. Don't expect your professional colleagues to understand what you did in the field—unless they are disaster trained, field experienced, and insightful to the craft. Even then, disaster tourism pervades the professional world and masquerades as disaster expertise.
9. Make time for an intimate partner—in a neutral area away from the domestic "real world". Both partners have paid a price for separation. Don't assume you fully understand each other. Give peace a chance.
10. Reach out to your friends, but lower your expectations. Your recent experiences can disconnect you from even your best friends.
11. Reach out to a mentor who knows you well and knows the field. He/she can help you process your experience. Those relationships can be among the most rewarding of your life.
12. Remember the concept of the 7 schedules. Reestablish the habits you found relaxing before your mission.
13. If you experience difficulty with reentry, avoid provocative agents—alcohol and illicit drugs. Seek support from someone you like and trust over a cup of coffee (in decreasing order of helpfulness: someone on your mission > someone who works for the parent organization > someone who has worked in the country of assignment > someone familiar with the region).
14. If you don't find support from the above, seek referral to an expert in adjustment disorders. The management principles are well-worked out, and outcomes from early referral are good.

Epilogue

Disasters do terrible things to people and societies. Survivors experience tremendous burdens but nonetheless typically conduct themselves with remarkable forbearance, resilience, and grace. They accomplish extraordinary things.

Health professionals have the privilege of assisting disaster survivors return to marginal self-sufficiency. There are many dedicated health professionals who have fashioned a career in disaster relief. Some careerists have distinguished themselves by advancing selected disaster best practices. A few superbly competent leaders, with inter-disciplinary, inter-agency, and international expertise, have pioneered the modern profession of humanitarian health assistance. They are the masters of the craft.

Frederick "Skip" M. Burkle

Skip trained in pediatrics, emergency medicine, and psychiatry. He has led the development of disaster health sciences as a professional discipline. He has advanced the field as an adept practitioner, prolific author, innovative program builder, and esteemed mentor to a generation of health professionals. He possesses three cardinal attributes of disaster health professionals:

- interdisciplinary expertise—triple specialty certified in emergency medicine, pediatrics, and pediatric emergency medicine with cross-training in psychiatry, public health, humanitarian assistance, and tropical medicine;
- interagency expertise—worked in governmental, non-governmental, Red Cross and UN organizations;
- international expertise—worked in over 30 countries including 5 major wars and multiple conflicts.

Among his landmark contributions, he authored the first multidisciplinary textbook of disaster medicine. He directed the first civil-military study center devoted to disaster management and humanitarian assistance. He pioneered the domains of civil-military cooperation and inter-agency technical liaison. For all his contributions, he was elected to the Institute of Medicine of the US National Academy of Sciences. In telling truth to the occupying power during the Iraq war, at both personal and professional cost, Skip earned the esteem of disaster field practitioners internationally and cemented his place at the apex of disaster professionalism. Skip is a visionary of the field and a master of the craft.

A.K. Siddique

AK worked as a bush surgeon for 17 years in sub-Saharan Africa. Field constraints commonly obliged refinements to his operative technique. For example, his generator-powered lights would fail after 15 min, so he mastered the 15-min skin-to-skin C-section. His patients didn't leak and their neonates survived. Nonetheless, AK found himself surrounded by public health problems that overwhelmed his clinical practice—epidemics among them. He gravitated to cholera epidemic management and eventually settled at ICDDR,B. With his unmatched corpus of experience in cholera endemic settings, and the science of ORS emerging at his institution, he became the world's foremost practitioner of cholera case management and disease control. His work with cholera treatment centers in Goma after the Rwandan genocide is legendary. Moreover, he was intolerant of distractions from quality care whether from inexperienced providers or egotistical academics. After *Lancet* published AK's original report on Goma, MSF wrote a letter to the journal editor in which it attempted to justify the high case-fatality rates of its cholera treatment centers. AK was unimpressed and deftly critiqued the excuses in a follow-up reply to the editor. When a self-promoting US academic made himself a nuisance in the field, AK acidly dismissed him as a computer hacker. AK is a pioneer in crossing professional boundaries and a master of the craft.

© David A. Bradt 2019
D. A. Bradt, C. M. Drummond, *Reference Manual for Humanitarian Health Professionals*,
https://doi.org/10.1007/978-3-319-69871-7

Judy Lee

Judy trained as a nurse and spent her career with the Red Cross movement. After growing up in pre-Castro Cuba, where revolutions alternated with hurricanes, she gravitated to disaster health services. She became the first nurse hired by the American Red Cross specifically for its Disaster Services unit. In nearly 20 years at National Headquarters, she served successively as Chief of Disaster Health Services and Manager of Disaster Logistics. Among her domestic contributions, she championed the establishment of ARC Disaster Mental Health Services. She innovated multi-site, multi-faceted service delivery to first responders and affected families in New York City after World Trade Center terrorism. She participated in the US inter-agency process that gave birth to FEMA, NDMS, DMORTS, and NTSB's coordinated response to transportation disasters. Among her international contributions, she deployed on numerous disasters with ARC International Services to Latin America and the Caribbean. She fostered the development of disaster nursing in the Caribbean as a consultant over 5 years to the Pan American Health Organization. Judy trained and inspired a succeeding generation of disaster specialists emerging from US academic medical centers by ensuring health delegate training and subsequent field assignments to enable their professional growth and development. Her awards include the Ann Magnussen Award, Jane Delano Award, and Florence Nightingale Award. Judy is a pioneer in disaster health systems development and a master of the craft.

Thomas S. Durant

Tom worked as a gynecologist and hospital administrator. His day job was Assistant Director of the Massachusetts General Hospital. His passion was refugees and disaster victims worldwide. While academic faculty at home hectored the outside world on humanitarian principles, and published self-congratulatory articles claiming influence on national policy, Tom was quietly serving disaster victims in the field. He excelled in mitigating the health consequences of armed conflict through clinical and public health programs. First the locals noticed, then the agencies noticed, then the international community noticed. His work with international organizations in cross-border settings helped establish the professional practice of disaster medical coordination. Among his enduring contributions are his rules of engagement in disaster relief operations. Tom cared little for recognition, but it came anyway—Man of the Year for the National Conference for Community and Justice, Humanitarian Award from the UN, and the first US fellowship in refugee medicine named in his honor at MGH. Tom was the archetypal humanitarian and a master of the craft.

Rules of Engagement

These masters of the craft are charismatic, observant, innovative, bold, and daring. They see and do things most health professionals cannot. Fortunately, they have identified their keys to mastery—rules of engagement—that enable others to best make their contribution. See following pages.

Skip Burkle's Rules of Engagement

1. Prepare thoroughly for your mission.

   If your mission fails, it will most likely result from lack of understanding of the country, the culture, or from inadequate team preparation and leadership.

2. Learn the local culture.

   Absence of cultural knowledge at minimum is equivalent to disrespect. At worst, it may be harmful to your patients and lethal to your program.

3. Learn survival language.

   Knowing the local language will make you less isolated, more effective, and may even help you survive.

4. Learn triage skills—for both patients and problems.

   A well-trained triage officer not only can manage a large number of direct cases but also will seek to identify indirect cases that may signal an emerging public health crisis.

5. Learn mental health skills.

   They will help you better understand your patients as well as yourself. Be an active listener. Listen more than you talk. Remember the most common presenting complaint will be a mental health one. A patient's mental health status reveals what trauma came beforehand.

6. Improve your physical diagnosis skills. Western trained clinicians rely on labs and X-rays which won't be available. Clinical decisions will be made on the accuracy of your physical exam and the "decoding" of vital signs.

7. Gather data on outcomes.

   We need to know and document health outcomes—what we did, why we did it, to whom we did it, and whether it did any good—in order to educate the next generation of humanitarians. Write up your experiences for others as well as yourself.

8. Schedule adequate time for sleep and leave. Beware of fatigue, drugs, and alcohol.

   Providers of acute trauma care should be high on your list for concern.

9. Establish personal friendships.

   Let these friendships be outlets for your personal and professional frustrations. While it's important to keep your own counsel, the more you can verbalize your frustration, the less harm you bring to your patients.

10. Master the three most adaptive defense mechanisms: resilience, acceptance, sense of humor.

    Stress management skills and coping strategies can improve the odds of a healthy outcome from disaster.

11. Provide leadership.

    Difficult or impossible leadership decisions will be the norm. Make them. But don't play God. Ask your team members for their input. Good, fair and shared leadership will result in better health outcomes.

12. Know how and when to delegate.

   Leaders may or may not make friends within their chain of command, but they must be able to delegate.

13. Practice humility.

   It's a good antidote to power intoxication.

14. Dare to be creative.

   It will be some of your best work. But don't promise or do anything that cannot be duplicated by the host country health-care providers after you leave.

Adapted by the authors from personal communication with Skip Burkle, Oct 11, 2016, and from Burkle FM. Coping with stress under conditions of disaster and refugee care. *Mil Med* 1983; 148:800-3. Used with permission.

Judy Lee's Rules of Engagement

1. Have a solid base of support at home.

   Reduce or eliminate worry over bill payments, schedule conflicts, and spousal separation, etc.

2. Travel to an assignment with as much information as possible.

   Ask questions about the type and scope of the disaster. Know what to expect and plan for it before you arrive on site. Mission essentials are: proper mission definition along with details of the disaster, assignment of key leadership personnel, and full commitment of resources required to fulfill the mission.

3. Travel light.

   Be prepared to carry your own luggage. Peanut butter and crackers may be all you get for a while.

4. Know the team members.

   Get to know any colleagues you don't already know en route or as soon as possible on arrival. Relying on each other will be key.

5. Be flexible—willing to work in an area of need that is not your original assignment.

   Florence Nightingale went to Crimea to care for war casualties and was assigned to medical supply.

6. Respect the work of others on the team not in the health field.

   There are necessary functions others fulfill in disaster management: accounting, human resources, logistics, etc. They are there to help you carry out your work.

7. See the big picture.

   See the whole picture to the extent possible—the whole patient, the whole family, the whole disaster. Women who do so will surpass those male colleagues who think only of finances, regulations, and machismo rather than humanity.

8. Keep notes on key issues and daily actions.

   A regular daily log will make reporting easier and preserve a record of actions you might otherwise not readily recall.

9. Teach as you go.

   Pass on disaster preparedness keys so that if there is a next time, mitigation can take place. You won't always be there, so help the locals to integrate and work with future incoming staff. Remember, they remain even after you leave.

10. Stay balanced in the field.

    Pace yourself, keep a sense of humor, make new connections, renew old friendships, get your rest, and detach periodically.

11. Know your limitations.

    Don't overextend yourself and risk becoming a part of the disaster rather than the solution. Be prepared to evacuate (others) and demission (yourself) as circumstances require.

12. Accept the need to continually train and prepare.

     Preparation is the best way to stay functional and indeed thrive in the stress of the field. Conferences, classes, standards, and regulations, including those of partner agencies, are within your scope of responsibility. You have to like the details.

13. Be able to sell your superiors on important policy issues when they cannot see the added value.

     Disaster mental health and disaster logistics were among the core concepts initially resisted by bureaucrats of the day. Involve the right people, compile the latest literature, accumulate data, and engage with your colleagues.

14. Read about inspiring and effective predecessors.

     Clara Barton, Jane Delano, and Florence Nightingale all changed the disaster world. You can too.

Adapted by the authors from personal communication with Judy Lee, Mar 3, 2017. Used with permission.

Tom Durant's Rules of Engagement

1. The purpose of the mission is humanitarian health assistance.

   Not data gathering for academic researchers, report writing for agency donors, or media relations for advocacy groups.

2. The work of the medical coordinator is beneficiary care.

   Corporate communications, accounting, and administration are all important, but if you are not directly serving refugees, then you are not touching those most in need.

3. Understand each other.

   Listen to people fully. Speak to people respectfully. People are sometimes the problem and always the solution. If you don't understand the people, then you don't understand either the problem or the solution.

4. Understand the complexity of refugee medicine.

   The best clinicians in refugee medicine know what supersedes their clinical work—most importantly, security and public health. You must understand those sectors in order to best run your clinical operation.

5. Don't re-invent the wheel.

   Read the work of your predecessors.

6. Don't make promises.

   When in doubt—observe, measure, and think (OMT). You can always be a good listener.

7. Don't sweat the small stuff.

   Wisdom comes from experience. Experience comes from mistakes. You will make them.

8. The biggest pitfall is arrogance.

   The best docs are able to say "I don't know", "I made a mistake", "I'm sorry", and "Thank you". Tom was hardest on himself. At M&M of cases from "unidentified" practitioners, Tom would publicly criticize his own clinical judgment.

9. The biggest asset is humor—even more than intelligence.

   Make friends and disarm enemies with humor. A joke on you is the best. Otherwise, Irish and rugby stories are preferred.

10. There are a lot of heroes out there. Find one and work with her.

    Most of the heroes are the refugees themselves, and most of those are women. They will generally be anonymous. Some of the ex-pat heroes in Goma were San Francisco fire fighters who provided clean water from pumper trucks, and Goal volunteers who buried the dead.

11. Stay the course.

    If you haven't been in the field for at least several months, then you are a medical tourist. If you stay long enough, you will experience predictable phases in your project. The classic ones are: enthusiasm, disillusionment, panic, search for the guilty, punishment of the innocent, then praise and honor for the non-participants.

12. Stay out of politics.

   Pinstripe is the most dangerous camouflage in the jungle. You need to understand politics but not to change it. Your job is to help your organization and its program beneficiaries—not to change the organization much less the health system in which it operates.

13. Do not be afraid.

   Any fear you face is likely a fraction of the fear refugees have lived with. Don't make a big deal about it. Get on with the job. If you are in a combat situation, then you may have to be a little brave. You do it 5 min at a time. Ultimately, you must anticipate, adapt, or die.

Adapted by the authors from personal communication with Tom Durant deceased Oct 30, 2001.

About the Authors

David A. Bradt, MD, MPH, FACEP, FACEM, FAFPHM, DTM&H

David A. Bradt is a specialist in emergency medicine and public health. He trained at academic medical centers in the US, the UK, and Australia as well as cross-trained in disaster management through the International Committee of the Red Cross, the World Health Organization, the United Nations High Commissioner for Refugees, and the US Agency for International Development's Office of US Foreign Disaster Assistance. His professional interest is disaster health services leading to disaster field experience in 25 countries and territories. Among his assignments, he served as emergency physician in the Mujahideen-Afghan Surgical Hospital at the Afghan-Pakistan border during the Afghan-Soviet war, International Federation of Red Cross medical coordinator in Zaire during the Rwandan genocide, International Rescue Committee physician in Macedonia and Albania during the Kosovo ethnic cleansing, WHO medical coordinator in Indonesia after the Indian Ocean tsunami, WHO emergency coordinator in Tunisia during the Libyan civil war, WHO senior public health advisor in South Sudan during its civil war, USAID/OFDA senior field officer in Sudan during the Darfur genocide, USAID/OFDA health advisor to the US Inter-agency Task Force after the Haiti earthquake, USAID/OFDA regional advisor in southern Africa during the El Nino drought, and American Red Cross medical consultant at US disasters including World Trade Center terrorism.

Dr. Bradt is a Rockefeller Foundation Bellagio Center resident scholar, a John Simon Guggenheim Memorial Foundation fellow, and a Fulbright specialist in public/global health. He holds a faculty appointment in the US at the Johns Hopkins Medical Institutions. He has served as senior health advisor to WHO Department of Emergency Risk Management, surge health advisor to USAID/OFDA, and medical advisor to American Red Cross National Headquarters. His awards include the Johns Hopkins Emergency Medicine Outstanding Faculty Award, Johns Hopkins University School of Public Health Society of Alumni Outstanding Recent Graduate Award for Public Health Practice, American Red Cross National Headquarters Volunteer Award in Disaster Services, USAID Meritorious Group Award to the Darfur Disaster Assistance Response Team, WHO Regional Office for South-East Asia Certificate of Appreciation for emergency response, Australasian College for Emergency Medicine Victorian Faculty Fellows Prize for medical research, and International Federation for Emergency Medicine Humanitarian Award.

Christina M. Drummond, AM, MBBS, DObst(RCOG), DTM&H, FRACP, MPH, MAE, FAFPHM

Christina M. Drummond is a specialist in infectious diseases and public health. She trained at academic medical centers in Australia, the US, and UK as well as cross-trained in disaster management and disease control through the International Committee of the Red Cross, the World Health Organization, and the US Centers for Disease Control and Prevention. Her professional interest is communicable disease control in disadvantaged populations leading to field experience in 24 countries and territories. Among her assignments, she served as Australian Red Cross medical team leader in Cambodia during the Khmer Rouge insurgency, International Federation of Red Cross medical coordinator in Zaire during the Rwandan genocide, American Red Cross epidemiologist in Guam after Supertyphoon Paka, International Rescue Committee physician in Macedonia and Albania during the Kosovo ethnic cleansing, WHO medical officer for tuberculosis in Indonesia during the Timor crisis, UNICEF-CDC technical advisor for Stop Polio in Sudan, CARE International health project manager in Sudan during the Darfur genocide, WHO public health consultant in the Maldives and in India after the Indian Ocean tsunami, WHO public health consultant in Cambodia after Mekong River flooding, and Medecins Sans Frontieres-Holland infectious diseases advisor for its projects worldwide.

Dr. Drummond is a Rockefeller Foundation Bellagio Center resident scholar. She holds an associate appointment in Australia at the Burnet Institute Centre for International Health. She has served on the Australian Civilian Corps Post-Disaster Recovery Team for the Australian Department of Foreign Affairs and Trade, National Tuberculosis Advisory Committee to the Communicable Disease Network of Australia, and Medecins Sans Frontieres Tuberculosis Club (international advisory group). Her awards include the Australian Red Cross Society Meritorious Service Medal, Australasian Society for Infectious Diseases fellowship, Association of Schools of Public Health research stipend at the National Immunization Program of the US Centers for Disease Control and Prevention, Australian Government Certificate of Gratitude for contributions to developing countries, Delta Omega Public Health Honorary Society membership, Malcolm Schonell Memorial Medal for contributions to humanitarian assistance, and membership in the General Division of the Order of Australia.

About the Society

The Disaster Medical Coordination International Society is a private, non-profit, operational, technical, humanitarian organization based in Washington, DC, which works to save lives through evidence-based best practices in disaster management and humanitarian assistance.

The Society endorses the following principled vision of health professionals in disasters.

- Professionalization of health personnel in disasters requires apprenticeship training, code of ethics, continuing education, and peer review.
- Qualifications for health professionals are competency-based, criterion-referenced, and time-limited.
- Competency is case-related—extensive field experience is fundamental to disaster expertise.
- Expertise in the disaster health sector is specialty-specific, site-specific, hazard-specific, and organization-specific.
- State-of-the-art in the disaster health sector emerges from inter-disciplinary, inter-agency, and international best practices.

Index

A

Anthropometric indicators
  adults, 178
  children, 176
Area food security reference table, 179
Assessment, 53–90

B

Bacteria, 207–209
Bias, 185–187
Briefing, 23

C

Chemical agents, 182
Chlorine, in water treatment, 174–175
Cholera, 227, 230–232
Chronobiology, 259
Communicable disease control,
       152, 225–246
Confounders, 189
Coordination, 141–150
Country and event-specific information, 2

D

Damage estimates, 87
Data collection, 56
Death rates, 189–190
Dehydration, IV therapy, 180
Deployment, 1
Diagnostic laboratory, in infectious diseases,
       152, 247–250
Diarrhea, 227–234
  clinical medicine, 230–232
  epidemic management, 233–234
  epidemiology, 228
  incidence, 228
  pathogens, 227–228
  preventive medicine, 228–229
Disasters, 1, 91
Disaster-affected population, estimation of, 85
Disaster-affected vulnerable groups, estimation of, 86

Disaster medical coordinator, 91, 141
Disaster medicine staff qualifications, 122, 139
Disaster relief operations, malpractice, 92
Drugs, see medications

E

E. coli, 228
Ectoparasites, 217
Epidemic preparedness and response, 152,
       221–223

F

Field assessment, 53–90
Field briefing, 56
  emergency management system profile, 39–45
  health system authorities, 48
  health system profile, 31–37
  medical handover checklist, 24, 27–29
  security checklist, 23, 24
Field missions, packing, 3
Field reporting, 107–120
  REA report, 107
  health situation report, 113
  health sector status summary, 119
Food and nutrition, 175-181
Fungi, 212–213

G

Gap identification, 88–90

H

Health care providers, 122
Health cluster meeting agenda, 141, 148–150
Health facility, 65
Health sector, 152, 167–190
Health sector status summary, 108, 119
Health Situation Report, 107, 113–118
Helminths, 214–216
Human resources, 93
Humanitarian programs, 152–162

© David A. Bradt 2019
D. A. Bradt, C. M. Drummond, *Reference Manual for Humanitarian Health Professionals*,
https://doi.org/10.1007/978-3-319-69871-7